S0-AJI-450

MANAGING CONTRACEPTIVE PILL PATIENTS

NINTH EDITION

by

Richard P. Dickey, M.D., Ph.D. (Pharmacology)

Chairman, Medical Advisory Board, Louisiana State Family Planning Program; F.A.C.O.G.; Board Certified Obstetrics and Gynecology and Reproductive Endocrinology; Clinical Professor of Obstetrics and Gynecology, and Head Section of Reproductive Endocrinology, Louisiana State University School of Medicine, New Orleans; Medical Director, The Fertility Institute of New Orleans.

EMIS, Inc.
Medical Publishers

Direct Mail Orders
EMIS, Inc.
P.O. Box 1607
Durant, OK 74702-1607

Telephone Orders
1-800-225-0694

FAX Your Order
(580) 924-9414

E-Mail Your Order
http:\\www.emispub.com

MANAGING CONTRACEPTIVE PILL PATIENTS
NINTH EDITION

ISBN: 0-917634-00-4

Published in the United States 1998

First Edition 1977
Second Edition 1980
Third Edition 1983
Fourth Edition 1984
Fifth Edition 1987
Sixth Edition 1991
Seventh Edition 1993
Eighth Edition 1994
Ninth Edition 1998

Second Printing - August 1998

This text is printed on recycled paper

DEDICATION

To Sarah

ACKNOWLEDGEMENT

My obligations to individuals and institutions who contributed to the publication of this book are numerous and only partially discharged by this brief expression of appreciation.

Special thanks go to my colleagues past and present who have co-authored many of the concepts contained in this book: Nichols Vorys, M.D.; Paige Besch, Ph.D.; Clyde H. Dorr II, M.D.; Sergio Stone, M.D.; Jane Weems Chihal, M.D., Ph.D.; Richard Peppler, Ph.D.; Steven N. Taylor, M.D.; Phillip H. Rye, M.D.; and Peter Lu, M.D.

A very special thank-you is extended to Louise B. Tyrer, M.D. for her contribution of the section "Teenagers and OCs."

Special thanks also go to my office manager Susie White, Gwen Wiggins, the rest of the staff of the Fertility Institute of New Orleans and to Lynda Blake, Mark Gibson, Susan Guymon, Pam Savage, and Debbie Weaver, the staff of EMIS, Inc.

TABLE OF CONTENTS

TABLES

Preface

The second printing of the ninth edition of *Managing Contraceptive Pill Patients* coincides with the introduction of a unique new combination 20 mcg estrogen OC, Mircette™. Mircette™ differs from previous OCs in that 10 mcg's of estrogen are given for the last five of the seven progestin-free days. This change has the potential to reduce breakthrough bleeding that has been a problem with 20 mcg estrogen OCs in the past.

In the first printing of the ninth edition, 10 new OCs were introduced, including two new low-dose formulations, Alesse®, a combination OC with 20 mcg estrogen, and Estrostep®, a triphasic OC with an estrogen dose that increases from 20 to 35 mcg.

Important findings regarding two major concerns about OCs have been published since the first printing of the eighth edition. New information about OCs and breast cancer indicates that a small increase in the incidence of breast cancer detected while OCs are being used is balanced by a higher survival rate due to the earlier stage at which the cancer is discovered and by the finding that cancer spread beyond the axillary nodes is decreased by at least 20 percent for up to 20 years after OCs are discontinued (Ref 65). This protective effect may be similar to that of having a baby before age 30. New information about the relationship of OCs containing the third- (actually fourth- [see Section #3]) generation progestins, desogestrel and gestodene, indicates that a widely publicized increase in venous thromboembolism (VTE) was mainly due to patient selection. The rate of VTE with third-generation progestins was not different from the increased rates seen for other progestins, including second-generation progestins when these were first introduced (Ref 395). Studies with this bias removed show that the odds ratio (OR) for VTE between third- and second-generation progestins was about 2.0, whereas the OR for myocardial infarction (MI) was 0.27. For both second- and third-generation OCs, the risk of death from VTE was less (one-fourth to one-half) than the background risk of death from VTE in women ages 15 to 44 who did not use OCs (Ref 273).

The latest information indicates that, for nonsmokers who use sub-50 mcg ethinyl estradiol OCs and who have no other risk factors (e.g., hypertension, obesity, family history of CVD), there is no increase in MI or cerebrovascular accidents either while using OCs or after discontinuing them. Although Leiden factor V mutation has been found to increase the incidence of VTE 30-fold in OC users and eightfold in nonusers, its incidence is low, just four percent of northern European women. Leiden factor V mutation causes resistance to activated protein C anticoagulant (APC). A report that APC resistance is more pronounced with third- than with second-generation progestins (Ref 350) has not been confirmed by other studies (Ref 395).

In this ninth edition of *Managing Contraceptive Pill Patients*, the sections on cardiovascular disease, drug interactions, emergency contraception, therapeutic uses of OCs and the subsections on amenorrhea, breast cancer, diabetes, epilepsy, gynecologic cancers, migraine, and nursing mothers have been extensively revised. Table 6 has been updated with new information about the effect of the third-generation progestin OCs on serum lipids. A triphasic OC containing norgestimate (Tri-Cyclen®), which has been approved by the FDA for the treatment of acne, is reviewed (Ref 337). This OC joins several combination OCs traditionally used for this purpose (see Section #15). Also, the section on drug interactions with OCs has been updated, using information from recent reviews on this subject (Ref 132, 375). Altogether, 156 references have been added to this ninth edition.

The effects of an OC on the body depend on the balance between the progestational and androgenic activities of the progestin and the activity of the estrogen components. Thromboembolic problems occur with OCs that have an excess of estrogenic compared to progestational activity. Thromboembolic problems have been reported in Europe for gestodene, which is the most potent of the new progestins and consequently is used at the lowest ratio vis a vis estrogen.

As in all previous editions, two principles of OC use are emphasized: (1) patients are different in their responses to OCs and (2) OCs are different in their steroid contents and, therefore, in the reactions they elicit in patients. Oral contraceptive pills should be prescribed on the same scientific basis with regard to their different steroid contents, as is used for other classes of drugs. Uniform labeling, however, prohibits such product-specific information. It was out of a need for such information that the first edition of *Managing Contraceptive Pill Patients* was written in 1977. That edition contained material originally published in 1969 in *Obstetrics and Gynecology* as an article, "Oral Contraceptives: Selection of the Proper Pill" (Ref 87). In that article, the side effects of oral contraceptives were organized for the first time according to their associations with either the estrogen or progestin component of the pill. Additionally, OCs were ranked according to their relative estrogenic or progestational potencies on the basis of their clinical effects rather than on milligram dose.

Major revisions of the original paper were published in 1972 and 1974 in the *American College of Obstetrics and Gynecology* publication "Seminar in Family Planning" (Ref 83). In these revisions, side effects were further organized into progestational, androgenic, and estrogenic effects and the biological and pharmacological effects of the individual progestins and estrogens used in OCs were catalogued. Using this information, it became possible to rank OCs on the basis of four distinct characteristics, i.e., their estrogenic, progestational, androgenic, and endometrial activities.

Additionally, it was found that, due to large variations in biological activities, the type of progestin was more important than the dose in determining progestational activity. Furthermore, progestins were found to have androgenic and estrogenic activities in addition to their progestational activities. In 1975, the author and colleagues produced proof, via animal studies, that the progestin component of OCs could either add to or subtract from the estrogenic activity of the estrogen component (Ref 59, 86). In 1976, the search for a more accurate method of reporting progestational potency was ended when a review of the methods then available found that purely progestational effects were separable from endometrial effects and that the latter were the result of the combined progestational, estrogenic, and androgenic potencies of OCs (Ref 89).

The first edition of *Managing Contraceptive Pill Patients*, published in 1977, brought this work together. For the first time, a logical plan for selecting an initial OC was presented, based on the individual characteristics of both the patient and the OC.

By the time the second edition was published in 1980, the estrogen component had been clearly identified as the cause of thromboembolic disease and a definite recommendation was made that only OCs containing 50 mcg or less estrogen should be used. Also in the second edition, a recommendation was made for use of norgestrel, because, in addition to being the most potent progestin, it also possessed the strongest anti-estrogenic activity.

In the fourth edition, published in 1984, the recommendation for both the dose of estrogen and the type of progestin was drastically modified. The recommended starting dose of estrogen was lowered to 35 mcg. The recommended choice of progestin was changed from norgestrel to norethindrone and related estrane progestins, which are less androgenic than norgestrel.

The reason for changing from the recommendation of a highly progestational and highly androgenic progestin to a moderate-progestational, low-androgenic progestin was based on four types of information.

The first and most important new information was the discovery that progestins suppress serum levels of high-density lipoprotein (HDL)-cholesterol, a "good" cholesterol that protects patients against atherosclerotic heart disease. The very OCs that were formerly believed to be safest because of their high-progestational and low-estrogenic activities were shown to produce the greatest suppression of HDL-C (Ref 38, 40, 219, 353, 500).

The second new evidence was that a positive relationship existed between the progestin dose and cardiovascular disease, as had been found for the estrogen component (Ref 20).

The third was evidence that progestins cause increased plasma insulin levels (hyperinsulinism) associated with vascular changes that could lead to atherosclerotic heart disease. This effect, although found for all progestins except norethynodrel, was most pronounced for progestins with high androgenic and progestational activities (see Section #13) (Ref 22, 125, 203, 256, 418, 459, 497, 499, 501).

The fourth and most compelling new information came from the updated Royal College of Obstetrics and Gynecology (RCOG) study of 1981, which found that the increased incidence of death from cardiovascular disease that occurred in current OC users was also present in former OC users for as long as six to nine years after OC use was discontinued. The relative risk of death from all cardiovascular disease was 4.0 for current users and 4.3 for former users (Ref 359).

Also, thanks to the efforts of scientists such as Dr. Swyer, originator of the Greenblatt-Swyer tests, the relative progestational potencies of different progestins were confirmed in 1982 (Ref 416) to be approximately the same as those reported by Dickey and Stone in 1976 (Ref 89). (These reports appeared in the first edition of this book.)

By the time the fifth edition was published in 1987, most physicians were aware of the relationship between progestational activity and long-term OC safety. In 1987, the uniform OC package insert was changed to include the information first brought to physicians' attention through this book in 1984 that increased deaths from cerebrovascular disease persisted for up to six years and from myocardial infarction for up to nine years after OCs were discontinued. In 1988 the sale of OCs containing more than 50 mcg estrogen was discontinued in the U.S.

In the sixth edition, published in 1991, the complete text of the FDA generic physician package insert was included for the first time. By the time of the sixth edition, the FDA had made two changes, one of which significantly affected OCs' prescribing. These were a statement that OCs were safe for patients ages 40 and older who did not smoke cigarettes and removal of the warning that OC use in early pregnancy might cause teratogenic effects.

The seventh edition coincided with the introduction in the U.S. and Canada of OCs that utilized the new third-generation progestins—desogestrel, gestodene and norgestimate. Desogestrel and gestodene have a more favorable ratio of androgenic-to-progestational activity and, as a consequence, lesser adverse effects on serum lipids than gonane progestins, levonorgestrel and dl-norgestrel. The biological activities of these new progestins were first introduced into Table 3 in the sixth edition, when their relative activities were not completely known, and were revised in Table 5 of the seventh edition. Many physicians switched patients to OCs containing these progestins in the hope that deaths from cardiovascular disease would thereby be decreased. The seventh edition also included expanded information on Norplant®, the first implantable contraceptive approved by the FDA.

The eighth edition of *Managing Contraceptive Pill Patients* included expanded information about Depo-Provera® injection, the first injectable contraceptive to be approved by the FDA. Depo-Provera® IM had been in use worldwide since the 1960s.

As always, judgments of healthcare professionals, based on knowledge of their patients' habits, individual characteristics, family histories and of individual OC characteristics, are the best guarantees that patients receive safe OCs suited to their individual needs.

R.P.D.
New Orleans
August 1998

Introduction

Popularity of OC Use

Oral contraceptives (OCs) are the most widely used and successful method of reversible birth control in the world. Since their introduction in 1960, the acceptance and popularity of OCs have continued due to their:

- High rate of effectiveness
- Simple method of use
- Ease of discontinuance
- Rapid reversal of effects after discontinuance
- Beneficial effects on the menstrual cycle

Risks of OC Use

The risks associated with OC use are low compared to the risk to life associated with pregnancy, except in women who:

- Have additional health factors
- Smoke cigarettes and are older than age 35 (Table 2)

Reducing Risks

Nearly all the excess risk of death due to OC use can be attributed to cardiovascular disease. It is now realized that the increased risk of cardiovascular disease continues for an unknown number of years after OCs are stopped. Both long- and short-term risks may be reduced if patients:

- Use OCs containing smaller and less biologically active amounts of estrogen and progestin, though this may result in intermenstrual bleeding or amenorrhea
- Are carefully screened and those at high risk advised to choose different contraceptive methods
- Recognize and report clinical symptoms that may precede serious illness early in their occurrence

Health personnel are often faced with the dilemma of choosing between an OC with high hormone activity in order to assure regular menses and continued patient use and an OC with low hormone activity in order to reduce side effects. The choice of OC must be individualized for each patient.

OC Patient Management

The essential elements to good management of OC patients are:

- Knowledge of the contraindications to OC use, both absolute and relative (see Section #21)
- Knowledge of the causes of common side effects (see Section #4)
- Ability to recognize potentially serious illnesses as soon as they occur (Table 12)
- Access to accurate information about biological activity differences among OCs (see Section #3)

Using This Text

Most of the known OC side effects and their causes are described in this text. Clinical information about the frequency of their occurrence and the usual outcome is provided, as well as a recommended plan of management. In many cases, the recommended course of management is to switch patients to OCs with different levels of activities in one of the four major activity categories:

- Estrogenic
- Progestational
- Androgenic
- Endometrial

Table 5 lists these categorical activities and should prove helpful to clinicians as they choose among OC types.

The activity profiles of various OCs are especially advantageous for the selection of an initial OC (see Section #21). The number of patients who can successfully use OCs can be increased if the initial OC choice allows them to avoid particular side effects; patients can later be switched to different OC formulations (determined according to their biological activity rankings) if side effects occur.

Recommendations for selecting an initial OC are summarized in Table 8. OCs listed in Table 9 are categorized into 13 groups according to their estrogen contents and progestational, androgenic, and endometrial activities. OCs from Groups 1-2 and 5-8 have $\leq$ 35 mcg estrogen and low androgen activity (less than 0.32 see Table 5), and may reduce immediate and delayed cardiovascular side effects.

It is estimated that 90 percent of all women in their reproductive years should be able to take at least one of the OCs containing 35 mcg or less estrogen without experiencing symptoms of menstrual irregularity and that 80 percent should be able to take these preparations without noticing side effects of any kind after the third cycle of use.

References: 81, 82, 115

NOTES

#1 Benefits of OCs to Reproductive Health

Non-Contraceptive Health Benefits

The following non-contraceptive health benefits related to the use of oral contraceptives are supported by epidemiological studies which largely utilized oral contraceptive formulations containing estrogen doses exceeding 0.035 mg of ethinyl estradiol or 0.05 mg of mestranol:

- Effects on menses:
  - Increased menstrual cycle regularity
  - Decreased blood loss and decreased incidence of iron deficiency anemia
  - Decreased incidence of dysmenorrhea
- Effects related to inhibition of ovulation:
  - Decreased incidence of functional ovarian cysts
  - Decreased incidence of ectopic pregnancies
- Effects from long-term use:
  - Decreased incidence of fibroadenomas and fibrocystic disease of the breast
  - Decreased incidence of acute pelvic inflammatory disease
  - Decreased incidence of endometrial cancer
  - Decreased incidence of ovarian cancer

-FDA Package Insert Labeling

Benefits of OC Use

Patients receive significant benefits during and after discontinuing OC use (Table 1). These benefits include:

- Avoidance of pregnancy-related complications
- Reduced premenstrual symptoms and menstruation-related anemia
- Reduced incidence of endometrial and ovarian cancer
- Reduced incidence of many common diseases
- Reduced incidence of gynecological diseases that adversely affect fertility

It is estimated that, for every 100,000 OC users, the following pregnancy-related conditions are avoided:

- 117 ectopic pregnancies
- 10,500 spontaneous abortions
- 10,407 term pregnancies requiring Cesarean sections

Complications of these conditions are the leading causes of maternal deaths in young women.

The beneficial effects of OCs on premenstrual symptoms and the reduction of anemia due to menstrual blood loss are well known but too often taken for granted. OCs reduce the incidence of fibrocystic and fibroadenomatous diseases of the breast and of reproductive cancers, including:

- Ovarian cancer
- Endometrial cancer

Additionally, breast biopsies are reduced by 50 percent in OC users.

An important beneficial effect of OCs for women who want to delay child-bearing is the protection they provide against four of the most frequent causes of infertility:

- Endometriosis
- Pelvic inflammatory disease (PID)
- Ovarian cysts
- Uterine fibroids

New cases of these diseases are reduced by 50 to 70 percent in OC users. These diseases account for approximately 50 percent of all infertility due to a female factor and 90 percent of infertility that requires surgical treatment.

Toxic shock syndrome is reduced by 60 percent (Table 1).

OCs are the preferred method of contraception in women who:

- Wish to delay conception
- Have not completed their child-bearing
- Have menstrual irregularities
- Are at increased risk of developing endometriosis

By comparison, the intrauterine device (IUD) has inherent hazards to health and future fertility, including a more than double incidence of PID; and barrier methods are associated with a markedly greater rate of accidental pregnancy.

Safety of Use

Combination OCs are equal to or surpass other contraceptive methods in safety compared to pregnancy until age 35 for smokers and throughout life for nonsmokers (Table 2). In April of 1990, the FDA ordered revised labeling for oral contraceptive products to reflect current scientific opinion that the benefits of oral contraception for healthy nonsmoking women over age 40 may outweigh the possible risks. An increased risk of cardiovascular disease that can be attributed to oral contraceptive use remains a possibility in this population. This risk, however, may be less than those associated with pregnancy and alternative surgical and medical procedures that may be needed should pregnancy occur. To minimize risks, older women should be cautioned to take the lowest possible dose formulation that is effective.

All of the increased mortality associated with OC use is related to cardiovascular disease (CVD), and most of the risk is proportional to estrogen and progestin contents of OC preparations. For this reason, OC use is safest throughout reproductive life in women who:

- Have no cardiovascular risk factors, i.e.:
  - Hypertension
  - Obesity
  - Hyperlipidemia
  - Diabetes
- Have no family history of CVD
- Do not smoke
- Use regimens containing an average of:
  - Estrogen doses of 35 mcg or less
  - Progestin doses with potencies equal to or less than 0.4 or 0.5 mg norethindrone

A further reduction of the hazards of combination OCs may be achieved with:

- Progestin-only OCs
- Progestin injections
- Progestin implants
- Progestin-containing IUDs

These methods are nearly equal to combination OCs in effectiveness but are associated with increased menstrual irregularity.

Reasons for Choosing OCs

The choice of a specific contraceptive method for a particular woman may change during her reproductive life due to aging and changing desires for additional pregnancies. OC use is the preferred method of contraception for most younger women because:

- OCs are the most effective method of contraception
- OCs reduce menstrual flow and dysmenorrhea
- OCs preserve future fertility better than other methods, including barrier methods and periodic abstinence
- The return to fertility after stopping OCs is rapid and does not require medical assistance
- OCs have a favorable record of safety for women younger than age 35 who do not smoke

The choice of a contraceptive method should be individualized for each patient and will depend on many factors, especially OC effectiveness and risks of serious side effects (see Sections #2, #4, #19, and #21).

References: 42, 43, 56, 61, 109, 110, 146, 190, 205, 209, 242, 303, 304, 305, 306, 308, 330, 331, 356, 358, 374, 381, 382, 460, 461, 473, 477, 478, 482, 505

#2 Composition and Effectiveness

OC Composition

Oral contraceptives (OCs) have two possible components:

- Synthetic estrogen
- Synthetic progestin (a compound with progestational properties)

Two synthetic estrogen and 12 synthetic progestin possibilities are available, although not all progestins are available in all countries. Estrogens and progestins vary in their biological activities (Table 3).

The compositions and identifying characteristics of OCs available in the U.S. are shown in Table 4. OCs also contain inactive ingredients that act as fillers and preservatives. Rarely, patients are allergic to nonsteroidal contents (shown in footnotes of Table 4). When an allergic reaction occurs, it is most often due to lactose. There are eight OCs, all monophasics, that do not contain lactose.

Available OCs may be classified by type as:

- Combination OCs
- Biphasic OCs
- Triphasic OCs
- Sequential OCs
- Progestin-only OCs

In combination OCs, the types and doses of estrogen and progestin remain constant during the 21 days that tablets are taken, though the doses and ratios of estrogens and progestins vary from one preparation to another. Many combination OCs are also available in 28-day packages, some of which contain seven ferrous fumarate or inert tablets.

In biphasic and triphasic OCs, the dose of the progestin or estrogen component changes during the cycle in an effort to duplicate the pattern of the ovulatory menstrual cycle. Packs for 21 or 28 days are available; 28-day preparations include seven inert tablets.

Sequential preparations have been discontinued in the U.S. and Canada because of possible increased risks of adverse reactions, including endometrial cancer. These regimens included 14 to 15 days of estrogen in doses above 50 mcg, followed by five to six days of estrogen and progestin.

Progestin-only OCs contain no estrogen and are taken continuously. They are available in 28- to 42-day packages.

Dose and Ratio of Estrogen and Progestin

Estrogen doses in OCs have ranged from 20 to 150 mcg. Since 1988 doses greater than 50 mcg have not been sold in the U.S. Progestin doses as high as 10 mg have been used in the past in combination OCs and from 0.05 to 1 mg in multiphasic OCs.

In the U.S. combination OCs now contain 0.1 to 1 mg of progestin. Progestin-only preparations may contain as little as 0.075 mg, and progestin and triphasic preparations may contain as little as 0.05 mg progestin on some days.

The ratio of estrogen-to-progestin in combination OCs ranges from 1:5 to 1:50, with the most commonly prescribed OCs having a ratio of 1:10 to 1:30.

In the normal menstrual cycle, the ratio of active serum estrogen (estradiol plus estrone)-to-progesterone averages:

- 1:10 during the early follicular phase
- 1:5 during the pre-ovulatory phase
- 1:50 during the luteal phase

Multiphasic OCs attempt to duplicate these ratios cyclically by varying the doses or progestin and estrogen.

OC Effectiveness

Contraceptive activity can result from either the estrogen or progestin component. Progestin-only and combination OCs containing very low doses of estrogen have slightly reduced effectiveness.

Contraceptive activity results from:

- Prevention of ovulation by suppression of hypothalamic and pituitary secretions (due to estrogenic and progestational actions)
- Alteration of cervical mucus to make it hostile to sperm (due to progestational and androgenic actions)
- Alteration of endometrial lining, preventing implantation (due to androgenic, estrogenic, and progestational actions)

Pregnancy while taking OCs may be due to:

- Method failure (lack of OC efficacy)
- Patient failure (omission of OCs)
- Concurrent use of other drugs (see Section #5)

It is especially important that patients be advised not to omit taking OCs when low-dose formulations are used.

Most failures are due to patient error in the first months of OC use. For this reason, many practitioners advise patients to use concurrent backup contraception with the first packs of OCs (see Section #19).

Contraceptive effectiveness is expressed as the Pearl Index. This indicates the number of pregnancies that occur for every 1,200 cycles, or 100 women per years of use.

There is no significant difference in combined failure rates between OCs containing 20 to 35 mcg of estrogen and those containing 50 mcg, according to manufacturer's data submitted to the FDA at the time of new drug applications. The combined failure rate is that due to all causes. Combined failure rates are:

- 0.79 for OCs with 20 mcg estrogen
- 0.13 to 1.3 for OCs with 30 to 35 mcg estrogen
- 0.08 to 0.88 for OCs with 50 mcg estrogen

The differences in these reported failure rates are too small to justify using estrogen doses higher than 20 to 35 mcg even when highest contraceptive effectiveness is desired.

Family planning programs that have conducted independent studies show combination and multiphasic OC method failure rates of about 2.0. This is higher than the rate reported by manufacturers. The combined pregnancy rate for OCs containing progestin only is 2.3 to 2.5. Some clinicians believe that the accidental omission of an OC may be more likely to result in pregnancy when low-dose combination or progestin-only OCs are used.

Different manufacturing processes may result in different potencies of generic OCs with the same stated dosages. The efficacy of generic OCs may not equal that of established products with similar doses. The FDA requires only that generic OCs have 75 percent of the estrogen and progestin contained in name-brand OCs.

Lack of effectiveness could be critical for low-dose generic OCs that meet only the minimal FDA standards. Generic OCs that contain 50 mcg ethinyl estradiol and 1 mg norethindrone or another progestin with equal progestational activity should provide contraceptive activity equal to name brands even with only 75-percent activity.

References: 83, 87, 143

#3 Comparative Activities of OCs

Types of Biological Activity
Progestin Structure/Activity Relationships
Measurement of Biological Activity
Effect of OCs on Serum Lipids
Individual OC Activity

3.

TYPES OF BIOLOGICAL ACTIVITY

In addition to contraceptive activity or efficacy (see Section #2), OCs have five major types of biological activities. These are:
- Estrogenic activity
- Progestational activity
- Androgenic activity
- Endometrial activity
- Effect on serum lipoproteins

Table 3 lists the biological activities of individual contraceptive components (estrogens and progestins); Table 5 lists the biological activities of individual OCs.

The biological activity of an OC is a result of the combined activities of the estrogen and progestin components. Because of differences in the makeup of these components, each OC formulation has a different pattern of biological activity. The results of the estrogenic, progestational, and androgenic activities may be seen in the side effects that occur when an excess or deficiency of one of the steroid components occurs (Table 11) and in effects on serum lipids (Table 6).

PROGESTIN STRUCTURE/ ACTIVITY RELATIONSHIPS

Most progestins used in the original OCs, introduced in the early 1960s were structurally similar to androgens, except that they lacked a methyl (CH_3) group at the 19 position. The term 19-nor-progestin was used to describe these compounds, and they were named, as a group, the estrane progestins.

The first-generation (I) 19-nor-progestins (norethindrone [norethisterone]) contained only this change, plus the addition of an ethinyl group at the 17 position, which markedly increases the activity of any steroids taken orally. Norethynodrel, the first 19-nor-progestins to be employed in an OC (Enovid®), had in common with estrogens a double-bond between the five and 10 positions (between the A and B rings) rather than between the four and five positions. As a result, norethynodrel, unlike norethindrone (norethisterone), had no androgenic activity and had more estrogenic activity than other 19-nor-progestins.

The second-generation (II) of OC progestins were estrane compounds to which acetate groups were added at the 17 position (norethindrone acetate [norethisterone acetate]) or at both the 17 and three positions (ethynodiol diacetate or ethynodrel diacetate). Both of these additions increased overall progestational activity. Androgenic activity was increased by the acetate at the 17 position (norethindrone acetate) and decreased by an acetate at the three position (ethynodiol diacetate).

In the third-generation (III) 19-nor-progestins, a methyl group was attached to the C-18 methyl group to create an ethyl group at C-13, creating the gonane group of progestins (dl-norgestrel, levonorgestrel). These compounds had increased progestational potencies compared to estrane progestins and were also more androgenic. In addition, they completely lacked estrogenic activity.

In fourth-generation (IV) progestins, the 13-ethinyl gonane structure has been modified further by the addition of a methylene group at the 11 position (desogestrel), the addition of an acetate group at the 17 position, and the addition of a nitrogen at the three position (norgestimate) or the introduction of a double-bond between the 15 and 16 positions into ring D (gestodene). The 11-methylene group increases the binding to the progesterone receptor and reduces binding to the androgen receptor compared to levonorgestrel. The 15-to-16 double-bond increases binding only to the progesterone receptor, while binding to the androgen receptor is unchanged.

- 5(10) Estrane [17-ethinyl, 19-nor-5(10) testosterone]
  - Norethynodrel (I)
- Estrane (17-ethinyl, 19-nor-testosterone)
  - Norethindrone (norethisterone) (I)
  - Norethindrone (norethisterone) acetate (II)
  - Ethynodiol (ethynodrel) diacetate (II)
- Gonane (13-ethyl, 17-ethinyl, 19-nor-testosterone)
  - dl-norgestrel (III)
  - Levonorgestrel (LNG) (III)
  - Desogestrel (IV)
  - Gestodene (IV)
  - Norgestimate (IV)

The actual activities of some progestins occur only after metabolism to a different compound (the active metabolite) in the liver and intestinal wall. Thus, estrane progestins are metabolized to norethindrone (norethisterone). For fourth-generation progestins, the changes to active metabolites are desogestrel to 3-keto desogestrel and levonorgestrel.

In those receptor progesterone binding assays that employ whole cells in order to include nuclear bindings, levonorgestrel is about 4.5 times, 3-keto desogestrel is about 8.7 times, and gestodene is about 8.7 times as potent as norethindrone. The androgenic binding affinities, however, are approximately equal for norethindrone (6.0) and 3-keto desogestrel (6.5) and are approximately two times higher for levonorgestrel (15.3) and gestodene (13.4) compared to norethindrone. The selectivity for progestational over androgenic binding compared to norethindrone was eight times greater for 3-keto desogestrel and 5.2 times greater for gestodene, both fourth-generation gonane progestins, and 1.8 times greater for levonorgestrel, a third-generation gonane progestin; however, the differences in progesterone and androgen receptor binding do not reflect *in vivo* activity.

Pregnane progestins have no inherent androgenic or estrogenic activities but may be metabolized to androgens and estrogens.

Both agonist and antagonist activities of contraceptive steroids occur at the cell cytoplasmic receptor. Steroids enter the cell by simple diffusion and bind to a cytoplasmic receptor specific for estrogen, testosterone, cortisol, or progesterone. Testosterone is usually metabolized within the cell to dihydrotestosterone (DHT) before binding occurs. The cytoplasmic receptor-steroid complex then translocates to the cell nucleus, where it binds to a receptor site on a gene in the DNA molecule. This results in the formation of an RNA messenger, which is transported to ribosomes in the cytoplasm. There it initiates the formulation of a protein that is responsible for the characteristic chemical or physiological action associated with the steroid.

Only the most potent steroids elicit the maximum response upon combining with the gene receptor. Less potent steroids and steroid antagonists may combine with the cytoplasmic receptor, thereby blocking more potent steroids; but they elicit no response or only a weak or temporary action when combining with the intranuclear gene receptor.

Estrogens cause the development of progesterone receptors within the uterus. Pregnane derivatives, such as MPA, decrease the number of progesterone and estrogen receptors by inhibiting estrogen receptor synthesis. Progesterone induces 17-ß-hydroxysteroid dehydrogenase, the enzyme involved in the conversion of estradiol to estrone.

The 19-nor-progestins have a steroid configuration similar to androgens but combine with progesterone receptors. A small part (0.25 to 2.26 percent) of estrane progestins are metabolized to ethinyl estradiol (EE) and then to estradiol. The 19-nor-progestins also act as antagonists of estrogens by one or more of the following mechanisms:

- Combining directly with the cytoplasmic estrogen receptors
- Metabolizing to weak estrogens, which then combine with the cytoplasmic receptors
- Suppressing the synthesis of cytoplasmic and nuclear estrogen receptors
- Inducing the 17-ß-dehydrogenase enzyme

Mestranol is metabolized to EE before combining with the estrogen receptor.

References: 53, 54, 157, 214, 215, 300, 320

MEASUREMENT OF BIOLOGICAL ACTIVITY

Estrogenic Activity
Estrogenic activity may be measured by either the mouse uterine or rat vaginal cell assay. EE is 50 percent more potent than mestranol in both tests (i.e., mestranol has 67 percent of the activity of EE).

Estrane and 5(10) estrane progestins exhibit weak estrogenic activities in animal assays. This activity is clinically significant because of the large amount of 19-nor-progestin relative to estrogen in OCs. All 19-nor- and C-21 progestins, except norethynodrel, exhibit anti-estrogenic activity or antagonism, which blocks some of the estrogenic activity. All progestins are inactive in estrogen receptor assays. Progestins, except norethynodrel, reduce the biological activity of the estrogen component of OCs. Estrogen and progestin components must be administered together in animal assays in order to quantitate the actual biological estrogenic activities of combination OCs.

References: 59, 86, 117, 197

Progestational Activity
Progestational activity may be measured in the human by the induction of subnuclear glycogen vacuoles. The number of progesterone receptors is dependent on the estrogen component. The ratio of estrogen-

to-progesterone receptors remains unchanged when estrogen levels increase. The delay of menses test (Greenblatt-Swyer) is not a specific test of progestational activity because the estrogenic and androgenic activities of progestins also influence the result. Binding affinities of progestins for progesterone receptors in the human myometrium are often dissimilar from their effects in the glycogen assay and the delay of menses test.

References: 28, 89, 111, 145, 149, 414, 416

Androgenic Activity

Androgenic activity is derived entirely from the progestin component; all 19-nor-progestins except norethynodrel have androgenic activity. The most common test of androgenic activity is the rat ventral prostate assay, with methyltestosterone as the standard. In humans, androgenic activity may be indirectly measured by effects on sebum production. Androgenic activity of the progestin in OCs is inhibited by the estrogen component, both by direct antagonism and by inducing increased production of sex hormone (testosterone) binding globulin (SHBG-TBG). The amount of circulating SHBG-TBG reflects the androgen/ estrogen balance of an oral contraceptive. If the balance is more androgenic, there is more unbound testosterone. This results in more androgenic side effects, such as acne, hirsutism, weight gain, and nervousness. If the balance is more estrogenic, there is less unbound testosterone with fewer androgenic side effects. Desogestrel and norethindrone depress SHBG slightly, and norgestrel depresses SHBG markedly. Progestins, especially norgestrel, can displace testosterone and DHT from SHBG. Additionally, androgenic activity decreases high-density lipoprotein (HDL)-cholesterol levels, especially HDL-2.

References: 20, 333, 422

Endometrial Activity

Endometrial activity is a result of the combined effects of estrogenic, progestational, and androgenic activities and also of the ratio of estrogen-to-progestin. Endometrial activity is best measured by the ability of the OC to prevent spotting and breakthrough bleeding (BTB). Changing the estrogen-to-progestin ratio by lowering the progestin dose may be useful in reducing BTB and amenorrhea, since both may be caused by a relative insufficiency of estrogen.

Endometrial activity is expressed in Table 5 as a percentage of patients who have spotting, BTB, or early withdrawal bleeding (onset of menses before last active pill has been taken) during the third cycle of OC use. These are combined, since the distinction between spotting, BTB, and early withdrawal bleeding is arbitrary and varies from one manufacturer to another. The occurrence of spotting and/or BTB is always highest during the first cycle of OC use, decreases during the next two to three cycles, and changes little thereafter.

Failure of menses to occur during the seven OC-free or placebo days is another measure of endometrial activity. Failure to menstruate is always due to a lack of estrogen stimulation of the endometrium, unless it is due to pregnancy (see Section #9).

Because OC manufacturers are not uniform in their methods of reporting failure of menses, their results cannot be used for comparisons of endometrial activities. Failure of menses is defined by manufacturers of OCs containing desogestrel, ethynodiol diacetate, dl-norgestrel, and LNG as the percentage of patients who do not bleed during the seven OC-free days. One manufacturer of norethindrone defines failure of menses as the absence of bleeding of any kind for 60 consecutive days (i.e., two full OC cycles). The manufacturer of norethindrone acetate defines failure of menses as the absence of bleeding for 42 consecutive days.

References: 83, 89, 439

EFFECTS OF OCS ON SERUM LIPIDS

The effect of OCs on serum lipids is the probable reason that the increased incidence of death due to cardiovascular disease (CVD) persists for an unknown number of years after OCs are discontinued. Studies of lipid changes caused by individual OCs are difficult to evaluate because the:
- Length of use is not uniform
- Parameters measured may vary with each study, with no consensus as to which are important
- Numbers of patients are usually too small to allow conclusions about the significance of results

However, there is general agreement that an increased risk of atherosclerotic heart disease (ASHD) is associated with:
- An increase in the ratio of total cholesterol divided by HDL-cholesterol
- A decrease in HDL-cholesterol levels
- An increase in triglyceride and low-density lipoprotein (LDL)-cholesterol levels

Recent investigations that focused specifically on the subfractions of HDL-cholesterol (HDL-2 and HDL-3) suggest that the principal abnormality of HDL in CVD is a relative decrease in HDL-2-cholesterol. HDL-3-cholesterol has no protective effect.

Although many serum lipid fractions may be measured and ratios can be calculated, measurement of HDL- and LDL-cholesterol (Table 6) and the ratio of total cholesterol divided by HDL-cholesterol (Table 7) are the only parameters for which sufficient data are available to compare the atherosclerotic potential of different OCs.

The effect of an OC on lipid metabolism is a reflection of the:
- Progestin component's:
  - Dose
  - Potency

- Inherent estrogenic, antiestrogenic, and androgenic properties
- Counterbalancing effect of the estrogenic component

OCs with higher ratios of estrogen-to-progestin or certain progestins, such as desogestrel or gestodene, have favorable effects of increasing serum HDL-cholesterol levels and decreasing LDL-cholesterol and ratio of total cholesterol divided by HDL-cholesterol (Tables 6 and 7). Progestins and OCs with higher androgenic activities or lower estrogen-to-progestin ratios have unfavorable effects of lowering serum HDL-cholesterol, raising LDL-cholesterol, and increasing the ratio of total cholesterol divided by HDL-cholesterol. The appropriate dose and type of progestin may reduce the risk for coronary artery disease. Combination OCs containing desogestrel or low-dose norethindrone are associated with the most favorable profiles. HDL-2-cholesterol (a good cholesterol) levels are decreased by androgenic progestins. In one study, LNG 0.125 mg significantly depressed HDL-2-cholesterol by 32 percent and a triphasic OC containing LNG 0.05 to 0.125 mg significantly depressed HDL-2-cholesterol by 10 percent but raised HDL-3-cholesterol by seven percent for no effect on total HDL-cholesterol. By contrast, low-dose norethindrone and desogestrel OCs slightly raise HDL-2-cholesterol levels.

The unfavorable effect of the marked depression of HDL-cholesterol levels seen with some OCs is mitigated because other components, such as LDL-cholesterol levels (which increase ASHD), are also depressed; the result is that the total cholesterol divided by the HDL-cholesterol ratio change is minimal.

A small elevation in LDL-cholesterol associated with use of norgestimate combination (+3.4 percent) and triphasic (+2.4 percent) OCs was incorrectly calculated to suggest a -0.2 percent decrease in LDL-cholesterol in a "review" underwritten by a drug manufacturer. By contrast, LDL-cholesterol is decreased by desogestrel (-2.1 percent) and gestodene (-2.5 percent) in combination OCs (Table 6). The clinical significance of small decreases in LDL-cholesterol is unknown; however, it is generally believed that a one-percent increase in LDL-cholesterol corresponds to a two-percent increase in risk of cardiovascular disease. The favorable reduction in adverse serum lipid effects of desogestrel and gestodene OCs compared with other gonane progestin OCs (norgestrel, levonorgestrel, and norgestimate) is partially offset by a small increase in venous thromboembolism (VTE) (see Preface and Section #12).

References: 3, 22, 23, 38, 40, 46, 137, 219, 220, 256, 353, 394, 471, 472, 499, 500, 501

INDIVIDUAL OC ACTIVITY

The clinical actions of OCs are based primarily on the activities of the progestin and estrogen components and not on doses, as some manufacturers have claimed. An OC's endometrial, estrogenic, progestational, and androgenic activities are dependent on the biological activities and the doses of individual estrogen and progestin components and by potentiating and antagonistic effects of one steroid component upon the other. The endometrial, estrogenic, progestational, and androgenic activity profiles of individual OCs are shown in Table 5. The effects of OCs on serum lipoproteins are shown in Tables 6 and 7.

References: 83, 87, 137, 219, 353, 394, 471, 500

#4 Managing Side Effects

Adverse Reactions

An increased risk of the following serious adverse reactions has been associated with the use of oral contraceptives:

- Thrombophlebitis
- Arterial thromboembolism
- Pulmonary embolism
- Myocardial infarction
- Cerebral hemorrhage
- Cerebral thrombosis
- Hypertension
- Gallbladder disease
- Hepatic adenomas, carcinomas, or benign liver tumors

There is evidence of an association between the following conditions and the use of oral contraceptives, although additional confirmatory studies are needed:

- Mesenteric thrombosis
- Retinal thrombosis

The following adverse reactions have been reported in patients receiving oral contraceptives and are believed to be drug-related:

- Nausea
- Vomiting
- Gastrointestinal symptoms (such as abdominal cramps and bloating)
- Breakthrough bleeding
- Spotting
- Change in menstrual flow
- Amenorrhea
- Temporary infertility after discontinuance of treatment
- Edema
- Melasma, which may persist
- Breast changes, such as:
  - Tenderness
  - Enlargement
  - Secretion
- Change in weight (increase or decrease)
- Change in cervical erosion and secretion
- Diminution in lactation when given immediately postpartum
- Cholestatic jaundice
- Migraine
- Rash (allergic)
- Mental depression
- Reduced tolerance to carbohydrates
- Vaginal candidiasis
- Change in corneal curvature (steepening)
- Intolerance to contact lenses

The following adverse reactions have been reported in users of oral contraceptives and the association has been neither confirmed nor refuted:

- Premenstrual syndrome
- Cataracts
- Changes in appetite
- Cystitis-like syndrome
- Headache

- Nervousness
- Dizziness
- Hirsutism
- Loss of scalp hair
- Erythema multiforme
- Erythema nodosum
- Hemorrhagic eruption
- Vaginitis
- Porphyria
- Impaired renal function
- Hemolytic-uremic syndrome
- Budd-Chiari syndrome
- Acne
- Changes in libido
- Colitis

-FDA Package Insert Labeling

Overdosage

Serious ill effects have not been reported following acute ingestion of large doses of oral contraceptives by young children. Overdoses may cause nausea, and withdrawal bleeding may occur in females.

-FDA Package Insert Labeling

Clinical Information

The steroid components of OCs produce effects in the body similar to those caused by the natural sex steroids produced in the ovaries. However, OC steroids differ from ovarian steroids in their:

- Pathways of entry into the main bloodstream:
  - OC steroids enter the hepatic circulation via the gastrointestinal (GI) tract and portal vein
  - Ovarian hormones enter the systemic circulation via ovarian veins and the inferior vena cava, bypassing the liver
- Blood level patterns:
  - OC steroids are administered as a single, large once-per-day dose
  - Ovarian hormones are continuously secreted in small amounts that vary throughout the menstrual cycle in the dose and ratio of estrogen-to-progesterone

- Independence of pituitary regulation:
  - OC steroids are not under the control of the negative feedback from the pituitary
  - Ovarian steroids are under pituitary regulation
- Duration of action:
  - OC steroid action is prolonged due to modification of the structure
  - Ovarian steroids have a shorter duration of action
- Biological activities:
  - OC steroids may include androgenic and anti-estrogenic activities
  - Ovarian steroids do not include androgenic and anti-estrogenic activities
- Action at steroid receptors:
  - OC steroids may react differently than ovarian hormones

Causes of Side Effects

Side effects occur when the hormone activity of an OC is either much greater or much less than the hormone effect of a woman's own ovarian steroids on:
- Reproductive tissues and organs
- Steroid receptor tissue
- The GI tract
- The liver
- Other body organs

Women taking OCs containing 50 mcg or less of estrogen usually have lower levels of the hormone acting on their reproductive tissues than they formerly received from their own ovarian steroids.

All women taking OCs have higher levels of sex steroids in the GI tract and liver, regardless of the OC dose, a situation which causes changes in many blood components manufactured in the liver (Table 10).

Classification of Side Effects

Parallels to nearly all side effects of hormone excess from OC use may be found in the symptoms and physiological changes of pregnancy. Parallels to the side effects of hormone deficiency can be found in the symptoms and changes of the pre- and postmenopausal periods. Table 11 contains a list of the most common side effects, classified according to their relation to an excess or a deficiency of hormone activity in the estrogen and/or progestin components.

A number of side effects are similar to those that occur during the premenstrual period of the normal menstrual cycle. If these symptoms occur while active OCs are taken, they are likely due to estrogen excess and fluid retention.

Management

The first step in management of any symptom is to decide if the symptom indicates the presence or potential development of serious illness (Table 12). If so, OCs must be discontinued immediately.

Some signs and symptoms may be potentially serious but do not necessitate immediate discontinuance of OCs. Patients with such symptoms may continue taking OCs for a short time while they are being evaluated. These symptoms are also shown in Table 12.

The second step in the management of a side effect is to identify its probable cause. The center index of this text groups side effects according to the body systems they affect:

- Cardiovascular system (see Section #12)
- Reproductive system (see Sections #9 through #11 and #26 through #28)
- Other systems (see Sections #13 through #16 and #29 through #33)

    Side effects are described according to:
- Their probable cause
- The component of the OC most likely to be responsible
- Whether the side effect is due to an excess or a deficiency of OC component
- Suggested means of management

The third step in the management of side effects is to make a decision about the probable clinical course of the side effect if OCs are continued. Many symptoms that occur in the first cycle of OC use (e.g., breakthrough bleeding and side effects related to estrogen excess) will diminish or disappear spontaneously by the second or third cycle of use as the body becomes adjusted to the altered hormone level.

Patients should be informed of possible side effects and instructed to report their occurrence. Patients should be told:

- Which side effects commonly occur during the first three cycles of OC use and should diminish or disappear spontaneously (Table 11)
- Which side effects may be serious and require prompt medical attention (Table 12)
- That their particular medical conditions or family histories make certain side effects more likely to occur
- That side effects are often unrelated to OC use

The fourth step in the management of side effects is to switch the patient to a different OC product that has a greater or lesser activity of the hormone that is causing the undesirable effect, if it has been determined that the side effect:

- Is of OC origin
- Is not dangerous
- Will not diminish or disappear spontaneously

Table 3 lists OCs in order of their four principal activities:

- Endometrial
- Progestational
- Estrogenic
- Androgenic

A switch to an OC with equal or greater endometrial activity can be made at any time during the menstrual cycle. However, a switch to an OC with less endometrial activity should be made at the beginning of the next OC cycle in order to reduce the likelihood of breakthrough bleeding.

The final step in the management of side effects is to allow the body time to adjust to a new OC dose or formulation. Two or three cycles should be allowed for the body to become accustomed to the new product.

References: 82, 83, 84, 87, 109, 110, 330, 331

#5 Drug Interactions

Reduced efficacy and increased incidence of breakthrough bleeding and menstrual irregularities have been associated with concomitant use of rifampin. A similar association, though less marked, has been suggested with barbiturates, phenylbutazone, phenytoin, and, possibly, with griseofulvin, ampicillin, and tetracyclines.

-FDA Package Insert Labeling

Clinical Information

Drug interaction is a major concern for OC users, since many patients take more than one drug simultaneously. Due to the length of time women take OCs, the possibility of concomitant therapy for coincidental disease is increased.

Drug interactions with OCs may be conveniently considered as effects of OCs or other drug therapies or as the effects of other drugs on oral contraceptive steroids.

The interactions shown in Tables 14 and 15 may:

- Reduce the efficacy of OCs
- Increase the side effects of OCs
- Modify the actions of other drugs taken

For patients well stabilized on OCs, the unexpected occurrence of breakthrough bleeding (BTB) or spotting may be the first indication of drug interaction. In such a case, OCs may lose their effectiveness and pregnancy could result.

Previously, antacids and isoniazid were included in the list of drugs that interfere with OC action or absorption. New evidence indicates that antacids do not reduce OC absorption. Although 14 pregnancies have been reported during use of isoniazid during multidrug therapy for tuberculosis, these pregnancies are attributed to rifampin, which was used concurrently (Ref 132).

Mechanism of Interaction

One drug may potentiate or antagonize the effects of another through:

- Interference with absorption from the gastrointestinal (GI) tract

- Alteration in drug metabolism
- Alteration of excretion of the drug
- Alteration in binding globulin in the serum (for steroid drugs)
- Interference at active tissue receptor sites
- Intestinal "hurry" by alteration of gut bacteriological flora

OC steroids, for example, are weak inhibitors of hepatic microsomal drug oxidation (i.e., microsomal hydroxylating enzymes). As a result, the clearance of other drugs may be reduced, resulting in higher plasma concentrations.

OC steroids also enhance glucuronosyltransferase activity, thus enhancing hepatic conjugating capacity. This results in an increased clearance and, thus, lowering of plasma concentrations of drugs that are ordinarily eliminated by glucuronidation.

OC steroids may also influence the use of drugs to treat disease states by altering disease processes. For example, serum insulin levels and glucose levels are slightly elevated by OCs.

Many drugs are converted into water-soluble degradation products by enzymes. The rate of formation of these enzymes can be increased by different drugs (Tables 14 and 15), including:

- Barbiturates
- Anticonvulsant drugs
- Hypnotics
- The estrogen component of OCs

One effect of enzyme induction is to accelerate the metabolism of the estrogen component of OCs. Rifampin selectively reduces plasma levels of progestin, while barbiturates reduce plasma levels of estrogen only. A secondary effect due to increased metabolism of estrogen is to decrease the production of sex hormone binding globulin (SHBG).

The liver enzymes responsible for drug degradation can also be inhibited by other drugs, thus leading to drug accumulation and potentiation of effects. This may cause side effects to occur at lower dosage levels of certain drugs (such as tricyclic antidepressants) in OC users than would occur in nonusers. Antibiotics may interfere with intestinal intraluminal regeneration of OC steroids from their sulfate conjugates, thereby decreasing their availability during enterohepatic recycling.

Vitamin C and cotrimoxazole increase blood ethinyl estradiol (EE) levels by up to 50 percent and, therefore, may result in an increase in estrogen-related side effects.

Both an increased and a decreased tolerance to alcohol have been suggested in OC users.

Management

Drugs that may reduce the efficacy of OCs are listed in Table 14.

Drugs whose effectiveness or tolerance may be affected by OCs are listed in Table 15.

Unexpected BTB or spotting may signify drug interaction. If a patient's drug use history suggests this possibility, the dose of OC must be increased or use of other drugs must be discontinued.

To prevent pregnancy, OC users who have taken other drugs concomitantly must use additional contraceptive measures for one full cycle after the other drugs are discontinued. Increasing OC dosages does not guarantee contraceptive efficacy and is the least desirable method of management. Failure of withdrawal bleeding may be the first sign of loss of contraceptive activity and may be due either to lack of estrogen stimulation of the endometrium or to pregnancy (see Section #9).

The potentiating synergistic or antagonistic action of OCs on drugs such as antidepressants and anticonvulsants may necessitate modifying the dosages of those drugs in order to maintain control of the disease state. A lower-dose OC or progestin-only OC can be prescribed or a nonsteroid contraceptive method used in this case.

When powerful enzyme-inducing drugs such as rifampin and phenobarbital must be used, it is recommended that patients use a method of contraception other than OCs.

It is also important to know which drugs are not affected by OCs. The activities of some benzodiazepines (for example bromazepam and clotiazepam) and some corticosteroids (for example fluocortolone) are not increased by OC use. Valproic acid is an anticonvulsant whose effectiveness is not decreased by OC use.

A full drug history should be taken from all OC users. Patients should be warned of the possibility of drug interaction and of the loss of OC effectiveness if they take other drugs concurrently with OCs. Drug interaction can be either an exaggerated reaction (intolerance and sometimes toxicity) or reduced effectiveness. Patients should be instructed to inform other physicians they may see and their pharmacists that they are taking OCs whenever other drugs are prescribed.

References: 1, 7, 12, 13, 14, 15, 16, 22, 23, 57, 70, 71, 83, 88, 95, 105, 109, 110, 121, 124, 132, 153, 154, 198, 199, 210, 229, 268, 275, 297, 298, 299, 301, 322, 330, 331, 341, 375, 391, 474, 475

#6 Therapeutic Uses of OCs

Menstrual Disorders
Gynecological Conditions
Hormonal Imbalance
Hormone Replacement
Other

MENSTRUAL DISORDERS

Dysfunctional Uterine Bleeding

OCs may be used in the treatment of dysfunctional uterine bleeding (DUB), a nonspecific term for:

- Intermenstrual bleeding
- Bleeding more frequently than every 24 days (metrorrhagia)
- Excessively heavy bleeding often accompanied by clots (menorrhagia)
- Frequent, heavy bleeding not due to organic causes

DUB is common at the beginning and end of reproductive life but may occur throughout reproductive life in some women. DUB may result from anovulatory cycles or inadequate production of estrogen or progesterone.

Irregular bleeding may also be caused by:

- Pathological pregnancy:
  - Ectopic pregnancy
  - Spontaneous abortion
  - Hydatidiform mole
  - A persistent corpus luteum cyst
  - Endometrial polyps
- Uterine or cervical cancer
- Endometriosis and adenomyosis
- Uterine infections (endometritis)
- Drugs that cause anovulatory cycles (phenothiazines)
- Use of anticoagulants

Medical conditions that may also result in DUB are:
- Hypothyroidism
- Hyperprolactinemia
- Diabetes
- Adrenal abnormalities
- Blood disorders
- Malnutrition

The diagnosis of DUB can be made by endometrial biopsy by pelvic ultrasound and often through use of a basal body temperature (BBT) chart. Treatment of nearly all forms of DUB can be accomplished with a balanced OC that has high endometrial activity. Some cases may also be treated with triphasic OCs.

Dysmenorrhea
Dysmenorrhea is often caused by prostaglandins (PG) released from endometrial tissue. When dysmenorrhea occurs without other menstrual abnormalities, PG antagonists should be used for primary treatment. Antiprostaglandins include:
- Ibuprofen (Motrin®)
- Naproxen sodium (Anaprox®)
- Mefenamic acid (Ponstel®)

However, when dysmenorrhea is accompanied by dysfunctional bleeding or when endometriosis is present, OCs are the drug of choice. OCs with high progestational activities are required for maximum effect (Table 5).

GYNECOLOGICAL CONDITIONS

Endometriosis and Adenomyosis
High-dose OCs were used for treatment of endometriosis and adenomyosis in the early 1960s and 1970s before more effective drugs, such as danazol and GnRH agonists, became available. Although high-dose OCs are no longer recommended for treatment of endometriosis, OCs with low estrogen doses are recommended for long-term management to delay

recurrence of disease, especially when preservation of fertility is desired. The severity of endometriosis is reduced and the time until remission may be increased by low-estrogenic/high-progestational activity OCs because they decrease the amount of menstrual flow and block ovulation. Epidemiological studies show that current use of OCs has a significant protective effect (relative risk [RR] = 0.4) against endometriosis (Ref 460).

Some clinicians advocate taking three packets of OCs (63 pills) consecutively in order to decrease the number of menstrual days (Ref 156). One study suggested that the incidence of endometriosis was increased in women who had stopped using OCs 28 to 36 months previously. If confirmed, women with endometriosis should continue OC use until shortly before they intend to become pregnant.

Fibrocystic Breast Disease and Uterine Leiomyomas

Fibrocystic breast disease and uterine leiomyomas are associated with an increased sensitivity to estrogen, as proven by their partial remissions after menopause. An improvement in both conditions is noted when low estrogen OCs are used, but the improvement is more impressive with the use of danazol.

Danazol has been approved as the treatment for fibrocystic breast disease at daily doses of 200 to 600 mg. A major drawback of danazol is its low contraceptive effectiveness. Additional methods may be required for effective contraception.

GnRH-a is also used for the treatment of uterine fibroids.

When contraception is desired, low-estrogen OCs are the treatment of choice unless contraindications exist. Medroxyprogesterone acetate (MPA) should not be used in the treatment of fibrocystic disease because of its possible association with breast neoplasia.

Ovarian Cysts

OCs are important in the management of many types of ovarian cysts. (A discussion of ovarian cysts that are found in patients already using OCs can be found in Section #26). Ovarian cysts discussed in this section include:

- Hemorrhagic cysts
- Simple cysts
- Cysts resulting from use of ovulation induction drugs
- Possible ovarian malignancy
- Possible endometriomas

Possible ovarian neoplasms that appear as cysts include:

- Serous cystadenoma
- Mucinous cystadenoma
- Cystic teratoma

Any ovarian cyst larger than 4 cm should be considered a potential neoplasm, and appropriate steps leading to laparoscopic or surgical exploration should be instituted. Vaginal or Doppler ultrasound (US) can aid in diagnosis. Cysts smaller than 4 cm that have no malignant characteristics on US may be initially managed by a trial of OC suppression. The best OC for this purpose is a high progestational activity OC such as Ovral® (0.5 mg norgestrel/50 mcg ethinyl estradiol [EE]) (see Table 9, Group 13). Cysts that do not decrease in volume by at least 50 percent (this may represent only a 20-percent decrease in diameter) after 21 days should be considered malignant until proven otherwise. Endometriomas will also fail to suppress by 50 percent in volume. Surgery is also indicated when endometriomas are present (Ref 71).

Hemorrhagic corpus luteum cysts may initially appear similar to endometriomas on US but will be suppressed by high-progestational activity OCs. They are often recurrent and can lead to repeated hospitalizations and possible ovarian adhesions. Recurrence of hemorrhagic corpus luteum cysts may be prevented by prophylactic use of combination OCs with intermediate progestational activity.

Simple cysts of the ovary usually result from preovulatory follicles that contained an atretic oocyte. These can grow to become 4 cm in size and persist into the next cycle. Simple cysts need to be differentiated from neoplastic cysts. Simple cysts are often recurrent and are more common at the extremes of reproductive life at a time when neoplastic cysts are also more common. Simple cysts should be treated initially with high-progestational activity OCs and then with intermediate to high progestational activity monophasic OCs (see Table 9, Groups 2-4, 6, and 8-12) to prevent their recurrence. In one report, 73 percent of adnexal cysts resolved during six weeks of OC treatment. Adnexal pathology was present at surgery in all 81 of the remaining patients (Ref 390).

Ovarian cysts are common in the cycle following use of ovulation induction drugs such as clomiphene and hMG or FSH. They may be either hemorrhagic corpus luteum cysts or simple cysts. Treatment initially is different from that used for spontaneously occurring cysts because, if OCs with too high progestational and/or estrogenic activities are used, follicle development in the following cycle may be inhibited. Therefore, OCs with intermediate progestational and estrogenic activities should be used initially.

If cyst volume does not decrease by 50 percent after 21 days, then a stronger OC may be tried for an additional 21 days. If the ovarian cyst still fails to regress by 50 percent, it should be treated as a possible neoplasm.

OC suppression of ovarian cysts can be started on the first day of menstruation in regularly cycling patients. OCs may be started at any time after ruling out pregnancy in noncycling patients.

HORMONAL IMBALANCE

Polycystic Ovaries

OCs are sometimes used in the treatment of polycystic ovary syndrome (PCO) (Stein-Leventhal syndrome). Symptoms may include:

- Excessive hair growth (hirsutism)
- Infrequent menses (oligomenorrhea)
- Obesity
- Acne

Other conditions that present identical signs and symptoms are:

- Insulin resistance
- Ovarian hyperthecosis
- Ovarian stromal hyperplasia
- Ovarian and/or adrenal neoplasia
- Late onset adrenogenital syndrome
- Cushing's syndrome

These conditions are all characterized by excessive production of biologically-active androgens and frequently are improved by OC use. The rationale of this is that excessive amounts of androgen produced in the ovaries are suppressed by the progestin component of the OC and that the sex hormone binding globulin (SHBG) production is increased by the estrogen component.

Estrogen stimulates the production of sex steroid binding globulin (SSBG), formerly called testosterone binding globulin (TBG). When estrogen levels are low, the amount of free testosterone increases relative to the amount of bound testosterone. Thus, clinical relief of androgen symptoms will likely occur when a moderate- or high-estrogen OC is taken, even though the production rate of androgen is unchanged. This positive effect of OCs is further enhanced when the estrogen is combined with a progestin that has low androgenic but high progestational activity, such as desogestrel, ethynodiol diacetate or gestodene.

When excessive androgen production is entirely of ovarian origin, sustained clinical improvement will occur with high-estrogen OCs only if the progestin component is strong enough to suppress the hypothalamic-pituitary axis. Combinations of 50 mcg EE with 1 mg ethynodiol diacetate (Demulen®) or 1 mg norethindrone (Ovcon® 50) are recommended for ovarian suppression in patients with PCO because of the high progestational and low androgenic activities of these progestins.

Decreased sebum production can usually be seen within one cycle (21 days) of OC use. A patient's failure to improve within this time frame is an indication that excess androgen may not be of ovarian origin. Patients with hyperthecosis or stromal hyperplasia, however, usually require longer treatment periods for suppression of ovarian activity and may not achieve such suppression at all. Suppression of hair growth requires lengthy treatment periods; reversals of abnormal hair growth may not be apparent for many months, if ever.

In one study, both 35 mcg EE plus 0.4 mg norethindrone (Ovcon® 35) and 200 mg spironolactone daily were more effective in lowering Ferriman-Gallwey scores than 30 mcg EE plus 1.5 mg norethindrone acetate; however, all three preparations were effective in reducing or eliminating unwanted hair growth.

When OCs with low estrogen doses are used, sebum and hair suppression may occur during initial cycles of treatment, but symptoms may return after three to six months. If this occurs, patients should be switched to OCs with higher doses of estrogen.

Patients who fail to improve after initial cycles should be re-evaluated for sources of androgen production other than ovarian activity. Patients who do show improvement should be allowed to continue OC use until such use is contraindicated by age (see Section #20).

There is no evidence that the pituitary or hypothalamus regulatory system is altered by continued OC use other than possible increases in prolactin.

After OCs are discontinued, patients whose menstrual cycles were infrequent or irregular prior to

OC use will usually return to their former cycle patterns after a few months.

Most patients with PCO will require ovulation induction with clomiphene citrate to become pregnant.

Hirsuitism

Hirsuitism in patients not using OCs may be due to increased androgen levels or low SHBG (see Section #12). One study comparing OCs containing 30 mg EE and either 0.15 mg desogestrel or levonorgestrel (LNG) found that both suppressed serum free testosterone by 60 percent, but only OCs containing desogestrel raised SHBG levels (Ref 309). Hirsuitism improved in both groups, but improvement was more pronounced in the desogestrel group.

Acne Vulgaris

Acne vulgaris (AV) is associated with ovarian or adrenal androgen excess. Menstrual cycles of AV patients often are regular. Treatment of AV with OCs should be delayed until one year post menarche to allow time for normal cyclicity to be established.

OCs used to treat AV must suppress ovarian testosterone and dehydroepiandrosterone sulfate (DHEAS) production and increase SHBG levels to be effective. If improvement does not occur, it may also be necessary to suppress adrenal androgen production with bedtime administration of dexamethasone 0.5 mg or prednisone 5 mg. OCs with a low androgenic-to-progestational activity ratio progestin (see Table 3) and high estrogen content are the best choices for treatment of AV. First-generation progestins, ethynodiol diacetate and norethynodrel (now discontinued) have traditionally been used for AV treatment. Third-generation progestins, desogestrel and gestodene, can also be used. Recently, Ortho Tri-Cyclen® (a triphasic norgestimate OC) gained FDA approval for treatment of AV (Ref 337). In a randomized, blind, controlled study, patients who used Tri-Cyclen® achieved an average 51-percent decrease in the number of inflammatory lesions and a 46-percent reduction in the number of facial lesions compared to

35 percent and 34 percent, respectively, in the placebo group that used only cleansing methods. Investigators rated 83 percent of OC patients improved compared to 62 percent of controls.

HORMONE REPLACEMENT

Ovarian Dysgenesis

Ovarian dysgenesis (primary ovarian failure or Turner's syndrome, XO karyotype), with failure to develop secondary sex characteristics, is relatively rare. A diagnosis of ovarian dysgenesis should be established by chromosomal analysis.

Other causes of failure to develop sex characteristics or menstruate include pituitary and ovarian tumors.

When height growth has ceased, significant psychological benefits may be achieved by stimulation of secondary sex characteristics and/or menses. One method of stimulation is to administer estrogen alone in increasing doses until maximum breast development has been achieved or until menstrual spotting or bleeding occurs. At this point, the patient should be switched to a low-dose combination OC so that the risks associated with unopposed estrogen may be avoided and menstruation may still be allowed to occur.

Premature Menopause

Premature menopause (secondary ovarian failure) may be treated with either estrogen replacement therapy or low-dose OCs that have a neutral effect on serum lipids. OCs are especially indicated for patients younger than age 35. Causes of premature menopause include:
- Surgical removal of ovaries
- Radiation to the pelvis
- Spontaneous ovarian failure

Hormone replacement treatment should only be started for these women after the diagnosis is confirmed by high levels of follicle stimulating hormone (FSH). Because of occasional remission in spontaneous premature menopause, some clinicians discontinue hormone periodically for six weeks in order to determine if spontaneous menses will resume.

Menopause

The use of OCs for menopausal hormone replacement in nonsmokers who are in early menopause (younger than age 50) should be reconsidered in view of the FDA's 1990 revised labeling for OCs. The revision reflects current scientific opinion that benefits of OCs for healthy, nonsmokers ages 40 and older may outweigh the possible risks of pregnancy for women of this age group. To minimize risks, older women should be cautioned to take the lowest dose formulation that is effective.

In theory, progesterone and androgen are necessary, in addition to estrogen, to replace ovarian actions completely, since the ovaries produce all three types of hormones during reproductive years. Low-dose estrogen OCs meet this criterion and are also safe if serum lipid levels are normal and patients do not smoke cigarettes.

OTHER

Blood Dyscrasia

Low-dose OCs can be used in cases of blood dyscrasia, when it is desirable to reduce the amount of menstrual flow. An alternative method of hormonal treatment is the repeated injection of MPA in doses of 100 mg every two weeks. Treatment intervals and doses of MPA may be increased to 150 mg every three months and to 400 mg every six months.

Continuous spotting may occur in up to 50 percent of patients during the first six months of use.

Evaluation of Amenorrhea

Before the availability of inexpensive FSH and prolactin tests, administration of a cycle of OCs was often recommended in evaluation of amenorrhea. If bleeding occurred, intrauterine adhesions and genital tract agenesis were considered to have been eliminated as possible causes.

Hysteroscopic studies have shown, however, that intrauterine adhesions may be present despite withdrawal bleeding. Additionally, serum FSH and prolactin tests may be rendered inaccurate for up to six weeks after the administration of OCs.

The **recommended** method of evaluating amenorrhea is administration of 100 mg progesterone IM. If the possibility of pregnancy can be absolutely eliminated, 50 mg MPA orally in a single dose or 10 mg daily for five days will accomplish the same effect and can be used instead of OCs when monthly withdrawal bleeding is desirable. Oral MPA is not recommended for diagnosis if pregnancy is a possibility. MPA injections (Depo-Provera®) should never be used for diagnosis of amenorrhea because of the drug's unpredictable length of action. If bleeding fails to occur after 14 days of progesterone or oral MPA administration, serum FSH estradiol and prolactin levels should be determined.

Evaluation of uterine problems as possible causes of amenorrhea may be attained through the use of hysterosalpingogram and pelvic ultrasound.

Test for Pregnancy

Test for Pregnancy
   The administration of oral contraceptives to induce withdrawal bleeding should not be used as a test for pregnancy. Oral contraceptives should not be used during pregnancy to treat threatened or habitual abortion.

-FDA Package Insert Labeling

At one time, OCs and some OC progestins were marketed as tests for pregnancy. OCs and their component steroids should never be used for this purpose because:
- Other, more rapid and more accurate tests using antibodies for ßHCG are available
- If the patient is pregnant, OC steroids may cause congenital anomalies

- A false positive result will be obtained from patients whose secondary amenorrhea is due to:
  - Dieting
  - Exercise
  - Estrogen insufficiency
  - Menopause

References: 101, 109, 110, 156, 214, 309, 330, 331, 337, 460, 480

#7 OCs and Pregnancy/Lactation

Pregnancy During OC Use
Conception After OC Use
Lactation

PREGNANCY DURING OC USE

OC Use Before or During Early Pregnancy

Extensive epidemiological studies have revealed no increased risk of birth defects in women who have used oral contraceptives prior to pregnancy. More recent studies do not suggest a teratogenic effect, particularly insofar as cardiac anomalies and limb reduction defects are concerned, when taken inadvertently during early pregnancy.

The administration of oral contraceptives to induce withdrawal bleeding should not be used as a test for pregnancy. Oral contraceptives should not be used during pregnancy to treat threatened or habitual abortion.

It is recommended that for any patient who has missed two consecutive periods, pregnancy should be ruled out before continuing oral contraceptive use. If the patient has not adhered to the prescribed schedule, the possibility of pregnancy should be considered at the time of the first missed period. Oral contraceptive use should be discontinued if pregnancy is confirmed.

-FDA Package Insert Labeling

Effects on the Fetus

The most recent studies do not confirm earlier suggestions of an increased risk of teratogenic effects to the fetus of a woman inadvertently taking OCs during early pregnancy. As a result, the warning that formerly appeared in OC package inserts has been revised to recognize this fact.

If pregnancy is confirmed while OCs are being taken, OCs should be stopped immediately.

Pregnancy that occurs during OC use may be associated with an increased incidence of:
- Spontaneous abortion
- Ectopic pregnancy

Spontaneous Abortion

In one study, the incidence of spontaneous abortion reported among current OC users was 26 percent.

In the past, female sex hormones have been used during pregnancy in an attempt to treat threatened or habitual abortion, but there is considerable evidence that estrogen is ineffective for this application.

Ectopic Pregnancy

Ectopic pregnancy, as well as intrauterine pregnancy, may occur in contraceptive failures; one study reported a slight increase in ectopic pregnancies among OC users over nonusers. In progestin-only OC failures, the ratio of ectopic-to-intrauterine pregnancies is higher than for nonusers, because OCs are more effective in preventing intrauterine than ectopic pregnancies. A meta-analysis found a reduced incidence of ectopic pregnancy in OC users compared to nonpregnant controls (odds ratio [OR] = 0.19) and a slight increase in former OC users compared to controls (OR = 1.2) (Ref 277).

Malignancy

The use of diethylstilbestrol (DES), a nonsteroidal estrogen, during early pregnancy may seriously damage offspring. DES is no longer sold in the U.S. Studies have shown that female offspring exposed *in utero* to DES have an increased risk of developing a form of vaginal or cervical cancer in later life that is ordinarily extremely rare. This risk has been estimated to be approximately one to four in 1,000 exposures. Although there is currently no evidence that OCs enhance risks of a fetus developing this type of malignancy, daughters of patients who become pregnant while taking OCs should be carefully monitored for evidence of genital cancer.

Management

Patients who miss two consecutive periods should be advised to discontinue their OC regimens until pregnancy has been ruled out. The administration of progestin-only or progestin/estrogen combinations to induce withdrawal bleeding should not be used as a test for pregnancy.

CONCEPTION AFTER OC USE

Delay in Conception After OC Use

Compared to other contraceptive methods, there appears to be an average two-month delay in conception after OCs are discontinued, though some women will become pregnant without delay. No single cause for the delay is known; it may be due to several factors.

The percentage of women able to conceive within 24 months after discontinuing contraception is similar for all methods. One 1984 study found that, upon discontinuing contraception:

- The conception rate was 30 percent lower for OC users than users of other methods during the first month
- No difference in the conception rate existed for OC users and users of other methods by the third month
- Women older than age 35 had a higher degree of temporary reduction in conceptions after discontinuing OCs
- No difference in pregnancy rates existed for OC users and users of other methods after 42 months for nulliparous women
- No difference in pregnancy rates existed for OC users and users of other methods after 30 months for multiparous women

It has been recommended that patients allow one to three normal menstrual cycles to occur after they discontinue OCs before attempting pregnancy and that other contraceptive methods be used during this time.

Prenatal vitamins with 0.8 to 1.0 mg folic acid should be started prior to conception (ideally three months prior) in all women planning pregnancy.

Spontaneous Abortion After OC Use

There is no conclusive evidence that the overall incidence of spontaneous abortion, when corrected for other factors, increases when patients become pregnant during the first cycles after discontinuing OCs. One study by the Royal College of General Practitioners (RCGP) failed to find any increase in abortions in women who stopped OCs to become pregnant. Some evidence exists to suggest that triploidy and some types of polyploidy are increased among abortuses from women who become pregnant soon after stopping OCs, but the findings in this study have never been confirmed. Embryos with these anomalies are almost always aborted spontaneously.

Multiple Pregnancies

Multiple pregnancies have been reported to be increased after OC use is discontinued. This may be related to increased conception rates once thought to occur in patients with polycystic ovary syndrome (PCO) who stop OC use. Such a situation, if true, would be limited to the first few cycles after OCs are stopped.

Effects of Prior OC Use on Children

Several large studies found no evidence for increased chromosomal abnormalities or congenital malformations in children of women who used OCs within one to three months prior to becoming pregnant. One 1986 study found an increased incidence of neural tube defect in children of women who used OCs prior to conception. The same study found significantly more weight gain during pregnancy in recent OC users. In 1990, the FDA package insert was changed to read "extensive epidemiological studies have revealed no increased risk of birth defects in women who have used oral contraceptives prior to pregnancy."

Long-term follow-up of children whose mothers used OCs prior to conception found no significant difference in children of nonusers in height, weight, development, and intelligence quotient.

References: 30, 37, 48, 109, 110, 112, 126, 133, 163, 164, 167, 171, 174, 177, 178, 191, 204, 222, 231, 241, 250, 253, 277, 291, 292, 311, 328, 352, 376, 400, 464

LACTATION

Clinical Information

Combination OCs reduce the quantity and quality of breastmilk and reduce duration of lactation. Progestin-only OCs have a lesser effect on production of breastmilk, and injectable progestins either do not affect or may increase milk production.

OC estrogens and progestins are found in human breastmilk when OCs are taken during lactation. The possible effect of this on a newborn is unknown. It was previously estimated that an OC with 50 mcg ethinyl estradiol (EE) transfers 0.1 mcg EE per 600 ml of breastmilk to the nursing infant and that the progestin transfer is 0.1 percent or less of the daily OC dose. It is now established that, in the case of levonorgestrel (LNG), 10 percent of the agent present in maternal circulation gets into the breastmilk (Ref 377). A time-dependent decrease in maternal serum and increase in breastmilk levels of LNG has been observed (Ref 432). Once transmitted to breastmilk, LNG becomes accumulated with the passage of time, resulting in higher levels in breastmilk. The author concludes that infants should be breastfed immediately after the mother ingests her OC rather than waiting until two to eight hours afterward, as previously recommended.

Management

The World Health Organization (WHO) recommends no restrictions on the use of progestin-only methods after six weeks postpartum in lactating mothers. However, use of combination and triphasic OCs by lactating women may not be desirable because of the OCs adverse effects of breastmilk quantity and quality and the possibility of effects on the newborn. Progestin-only OCs and injections have less or no effect on quantity or quality of breastmilk but may affect the newborn. If progestin-only OCs are used, they should not be started until at least three days postpartum. For prevention of conception, it is doubtful if OCs need to be started before 14 days postpartum.

OCs may be helpful in reducing breast engorgement once nursing has been discontinued.

References: 109, 110, 141, 185, 196, 228, 249, 290, 277, 420, 432

#8 Teenagers and OCs

by

Louise Tyrer, M.D.
Vice President for Medical Affairs
Planned Parenthood Federation
Updated September 1993

Medical Aspects

Serious health risks from OC use are lower for young women younger than age 20 than for other age groups. The estimated risk of death from OC use among teenagers is 1.3 per 100,000 users, while the risk of death in childbirth for this age group is 11.1 per 100,000 live births.

Significant benefits from OC use include reductions in:

- Incidence of ovarian and endometrial cancers (continuing through later life)
- Pelvic inflammatory disease (PID)
- Follicular ovarian cysts
- Ectopic pregnancy
- Excessive menstrual bleeding
- Excessive cramps
- Endometriosis
- Acne vulgaris, including subsequent disfigurement

Assessment

Health professionals evaluating teenagers for contraceptive needs should:

- Obtain family health profiles
- Obtain personal histories, including menstrual patterns and frequencies of intercourse
- Perform and assess physical examinations and indicated laboratory work
- Counsel about risks of pregnancy vs various contraceptive options

It is advisable that clinicians assure that onset of regular ovulation and menses has occurred prior to initiation of OCs for teenagers. However, adolescent girls with oligomenorrhea may have significantly higher androgen levels than those with normal cycles. OCs may relieve symptoms of excess androgen and irregular menses in these girls and may ameliorate the later development of polycystic ovarian syndrome (PCOS). Oligomenorrheic girls may temporarily experience increased fertility or revert to their original oligo-ovulatory states when they discontinue OC use. In the latter case, these patients may experience problems conceiving and require an infertility workup and treatment.

Social Issues

Unintended teen pregnancy often results in the truncation of young women's education, thus limiting their opportunities to gain the skills needed to compete in society successfully. A teenage mother is more likely to be a single parent, to be divorced or separated, or to live in poverty than are mothers of other age groups. Although six in 100 OC users younger than age 22 will become pregnant during their first year of OC use, the failure rate is four times higher for those using condoms and six to seven times higher for those using spermicides. For these reasons, the majority of sexually active teenagers seeking contraception choose OCs. However, most teens could benefit from simultaneous use of OCs and condoms, since condoms also provide some protection against sexually transmitted diseases (STDs).

Management

Minors should be encouraged, whenever feasible, to consult with their parents with respect to OC use. However, services should not be denied when this is not feasible.

Compliance with OC regimens and intolerance of minor side effects, such as breakthrough bleeding, may be problems for this group. Therefore, closer supervision, with prompt adjustment of OC dosage when necessary, is essential.

References: 366, 372, 380, 388, 419, 429, 439

NOTES

#9 Breakthrough Bleeding and Spotting/ Amenorrhea and Missed Menses

BREAKTHROUGH BLEEDING AND SPOTTING

Bleeding Irregularities
Breakthrough bleeding and spotting are sometimes encountered in patients on oral contraceptives, especially during the first three months of use. Non-hormonal causes should be considered and adequate diagnostic measures taken to rule out malignancy or pregnancy in the event of breakthrough bleeding, as in the case of any abnormal vaginal bleeding. If pathology has been excluded, time or a change to another formulation may solve the problem. In the event of amenorrhea, pregnancy should be ruled out.

-FDA Package Insert Labeling

Clinical Information

Bleeding that requires use of a perineal pad or vaginal tampon during the time active OCs are taken is referred to as breakthrough bleeding (BTB). A lesser amount of bleeding during this period is defined as spotting. The distinction between BTB and spotting varies from one OC manufacturer to another; some manufacturers present only their bleeding statistics without including data on spotting (though this information is available upon request). Data on both conditions should be combined for comparison among products.

BTB is most common with low-dose combination OCs and progestin-only pills. It is the most frequent medical reason that women discontinue OC use. It occurs most often during the first cycles of OC use while the patient's endometrium is adjusting to a lower amount of estrogen and progestin than was present during her usual menstrual cycle prior to OC use.

One-third to one-half of all patients who bleed during the first cycle of OC use will not bleed in the second cycle. Bleeding continues to decrease until it reaches a plateau in the second to fourth cycle. The plateau is reached earlier when OCs with higher progestational and androgenic activities are used.

Bleeding that starts early in the cycle (before the tenth OC is taken) or that is mild and continues from the previous cycle is usually due to insufficient estrogen activity. Estrogen-insufficiency bleeding is also associated with failure to menstruate during the seven tablet-free or placebo days of the cycle.

Bleeding that starts after the tenth OC is taken is usually due to insufficient potency or dose of the progestin component. Heavy menses and menstrual cramps may accompany this type of bleeding.

An analysis of three clinical trials showed that women who smoked were 30 percent more likely to have BTB and spotting during their first three cycles of OC use (Ref 349). This differential increased with continued use and reached 86 percent in the sixth cycle. Although the incidence of BTB and spotting in the ninth cycle was low (14 percent in smokers and nine percent in nonsmokers), not reported but also expected would be an increased incidence of amenorrhea (missed menses) in smokers. Another study found an increased chance of pregnancy in women who smoked while using OCs (Ref 392).

Causal Factors

The most common cause of BTB is missed pills. However, BTB and spotting may also be due to the failure of the synthetic sex hormones in the OC either to provide adequate stimulus to the endometrium and its vessels following menstruation or to maintain the endometrium and vessels until the end of the active OC cycle. This may be due to:

- Inadequate amounts of estrogen and progestin in the OC
- Imbalance between estrogen and progestin components
- Insensitivity of the endometrium to the OC

Bleeding may also be the result of:
- Drug interactions
- Infection
- Endometriosis

In one study, 29 percent of women who had taken OCs for more than three months and who had BTB tested positive for chlamydia compared to six percent of controls.

BTB can occur after many months of OC use. Bleeding that begins after OCs have been used for six months or longer may be due to:

- Progressive atrophy of the endometrium
- An increased rate of metabolism of OC steroids
- End organ insensitivity or resistance (tachyphylaxis)
- Drug interactions
- Infection
- Missed pills

Bleeding irregularities occur more frequently with progestin-only than with combination OCs. Because of such irregularities, the discontinuance rate for progestin-only OCs is higher.

Nicotine and other components of tobacco may increase catabolism of estrogen.

Management

Small amounts of BTB or spotting are not harmful as long as the diet is adequate and the patient accepts the inconvenience. Since bleeding may denote a lack of complete OC efficacy, it is important that clinicians advise patients to use additional contraception until bleeding has completely ceased.

Bleeding may be a result of spontaneous abortion or tubal pregnancy in women who become pregnant while taking OCs. Additionally, bleeding (as well as pain) may indicate pelvic inflammatory disease (PID) or endometriosis. Thus, the possibility of pregnancy and/or pathological conditions must be eliminated by appropriate examination before a change in OCs is considered.

Bleeding may often be stopped by switching the patient to an OC with greater endometrial activity. Increased endometrial activity may be achieved with:

- Higher progestin doses
- More androgenic progestins

- Multiphasic OCs
- Higher estrogen doses
- Different ratios of estrogen to progestin

Switching to an OC with a higher progestational activity is indicated for early withdrawal bleeding but is also effective regardless of when bleeding occurs in the cycle. Switching to an OC with a higher estrogen activity is effective only if:
- Bleeding begins during the first 14 days of the cycle
- There is a continuation of menses
- There has been absence of withdrawal menses

The ability of a particular OC to prevent bleeding and spotting is dependent upon the:
- Type of progestin used
- Doses of estrogen and progestin
- Ratio of estrogen-to-progestin

In Table 5, the column labeled "Endometrial Activity" lists the percentage of patients who experience BTB or spotting during the third cycle of OC use. These rates are based on data provided by OC manufacturers to the FDA and/or the Canadian HPB and on information about earlier products published in medical journals.

Doses of estrogen greater than 50 mcg are not needed in order to achieve the lowest possible levels of BTB and spotting. Most patients do not require doses greater than 35 mcg of estrogen. Because of the potential long-term adverse effects of progestins and androgens on the vascular system, OCs with low progestational and androgenic potencies as well as low estrogen doses should be chosen over other OCs with similar profiles of bleeding and spotting. Switching to a different OC may provide improved cycle control without raising overall progestin or estrogen doses.

If bleeding continues after an appropriate switch in OCs, the patient should be re-examined for other conditions that may cause bleeding. OCs may have to be discontinued and other methods of contraception used.

New OC patients should be instructed that BTB and spotting may be expected during the first two to four cycles of use. Patients can minimize BTB by taking their pills at the same time each day.

Women who use OCs and smoke should be told that they have an increased risk of BTB and spotting, myocardial infarction, stroke, and pregnancy. OCs should not be used by women ages 34 and older who smoke.

References: 81, 83, 87, 89, 145, 221, 349, 392

AMENORRHEA AND MISSED MENSES

Clinical Information

Absence of withdrawal menses is the failure of menses to occur during the seven days between active OCs. It may also be called silent or missed menses.

Absence of withdrawal menstruation is most common in women taking low-estrogen dose OCs that have relatively weak progestational activities. Symptoms may first appear after OCs have been taken for several months either because tolerance to estrogen has developed or because of drug interactions.

Absence of menstruation may be accompanied by spotting or BTB during the 21 days in which active OCs are taken. Manufacturer's information about the incidence of absence of withdrawal menses for a particular OC may be misleading (see Section #3).

Causal Factors

The most common cause of absence of withdrawal bleeding is insufficient development of the endometrium and vessels as a result of insufficient estrogen activity. Interaction of OCs with other drugs may be responsible for low-estrogen activity (see Section #5). Absence of menses may also be due to pregnancy.

Management

All women who fail to have withdrawal menses should be checked for pregnancy before the next cycle of active OCs is begun:

- Pelvic examination may reveal a small uterus if the patient is not pregnant
- Urine pregnancy tests utilizing antibodies against the beta sub-unit of human chorionic gonadotropin (hCG) become positive between 10 and 17 days after conception, though some tests may give a false positive or false negative reaction if blood is present in the urine
- A basal body temperature (BBT) of less than 98° F(36° C) for two consecutive mornings is presumptive evidence that a patient is not pregnant
- A progesterone withdrawal test for pregnancy is of no value, since it requires the presence of an estrogen-stimulated endometrium for menses
- Pelvic ultrasound with measurement of endometrial thickness can help to make a diagnosis. Wall-to-wall endometrial thickness will be less than 3 mm in amenorrhea due to lack of estrogen stimulation. Endometrial thickness of less than 6 mm is incompatible with intrauterine pregnancy

If pregnancy is confirmed, it may be abnormal. Ectopic pregnancy is more common in women taking progestin-only OCs. If a patient cannot return for an examination or pregnancy test, she should be instructed to stop taking OCs and use a barrier contraceptive method until a definite diagnosis can be made.

Patients initiating OC use should be told of the possibility that menses may fail to occur even if they are not pregnant and that they may become pregnant if they fail to take their OC pills each day.

Changing OCs

Patients found not to be pregnant after adequate clinical and laboratory examination may choose to:

- Continue taking the same OC and have no menses
- Switch to a different OC with the same amount of estrogen but with greater endometrial activity by lowering the progestin dose or changing to a different progestin
- Switch to an OC with a higher estrogen dose (up to 50 mcg ethinyl estradiol [EE])
- Switch to a multiphasic OC
- Continue with the same OC and take additional estrogen tablets

If patients choose to remain on the same OC despite the absence of menses, additional contraceptive measures are not necessary unless BTB occurs.

The estrogen content need not be increased if a switch is made to an OC that contains a progestin with higher endometrial activity (Table 5). If the estrogen amount is increased, it should not exceed 50 mcg EE, since this level achieves the highest endometrial activity.

Amenorrheic patients taking a 20 to 35 mcg OC may take additional estrogen daily (Estinyl® 0.02 mg, Schering; Estrace® 1 mg, Mead Johnson Laboratories; or Premarin® 0.625 mg, Wyeth-Ayerst Laboratories) as an alternative to switching to combination OCs with 50 mcg of estrogen. The switch to an OC with a higher estrogen content or the addition of EE tablets should be contemplated only after attempts to restore menses by switching to an OC with higher endometrial activity.

A higher estrogen content OC should be used for only one or two cycles before returning to a lower-dose product. Continued use of higher estrogen OCs should be considered only after failure of all other measures to produce withdrawal bleeding.

References: 81, 82, 83

NOTES

#10 Heavy Menses/Dysmenorrhea

HEAVY MENSES

Clinical Information
Heavy menses, termed hypermenorrhea or menorrhagia, is much less common than decreased flow in OC users. If heavy menses occurs, however, it may be due to progestational deficiency and is sometimes associated with premenstrual bleeding or spotting.

Occasionally, heavy menses may be due to pathological causes, such as:
- Neoplasia of the uterus
- Uterine leiomyoma
- Adenomyosis
- Neoplasia of the circulatory system
- Abnormal pregnancy
- Endometrial polyps

Causal Factors
Excessively heavy menses, with or without clots, or prolonged menses may be associated with an insufficient progestational or excessive estrogenic effect. These symptoms are similar to those of nonusers of OCs who have anovulatory cycles. A delay in onset of menses until nearly time to restart active OCs is also due to progestational deficiency.

Management
Pathological causes must be ruled out by appropriate methods. To control nonpathological hypermenorrhea, patients may be switched OCs with greater progestational and androgenic activities and/or lower estrogen doses.

References: 81, 83

DYSMENORRHEA

Clinical Information

Painful menstruation (menstrual cramps, dysmenorrhea) is rare in patients with anovulatory cycles unless they pass blood clots or have adenomyosis, a form of endometriosis. Patients who experienced dysmenorrhea prior to OC use often note relief while taking OCs, but women who were anovulatory prior to taking OCs may begin to experience menstrual cramps.

The symptoms and severity of adenomyosis and endometriosis are decreased in women using OCs, especially low-estrogen and high progestational-potency OCs.

Uterine descensus, which may be accompanied by loss of urine, should be suspected if pain first occurs several months after starting OCs or worsens when patients stand for prolonged periods or lift objects.

Pelvic infection may occur at any time during OC use; it is often accompanied by:

- Breakthrough bleeding or spotting
- Increased or prolonged bleeding during menses
- Dyspareunia

The incidence of new pelvic infection may be reduced in OC users.

Causal Factors

The etiology of primary dysmenorrhea is unknown. Proposed causes are:

- Hypercontractility of the uterus due to release of endometrial toxins or prostaglandins
- Vasoconstriction
- Pathological changes within the sacral nerve
- Adenomyosis and endometriosis
- Endometritis and severe cervicitis

Other possible causes of menstrual pain are uterine descensus and infection.

Management

An examination is necessary to rule out possible pathological conditions. If none are found, menstrual cramps are usually reduced by switching patients to OCs with greater progestational and androgenic activities and less estrogenic activities. However, if symptoms are due to uterine descensus, pain may worsen.

Prostaglandin-synthesis antagonists, such as ibuprofen and naproxen sodium, are effective in relieving primary dysmenorrhea due to prostaglandin excess.

Uterine descensus may be diagnosed if the uterus is retroverted or low in the vagina due to poor support or if stretching the uterosacral ligaments elicits pain. Endometriosis located in the uterosacral ligaments causes findings similar to uterine descensus on examination, except that palpable nodules are often present. If pain is due to uterine descensus, switching patients to OCs with higher estrogen activities may relieve the symptoms.

If, on examination, the uterine fundus is tender, pelvic infection may be present. However, because the uterine findings in adenomyosis are similar to those of pelvic infection, additional diagnostic procedures may be needed. All pelvic infections should be treated immediately with appropriate antibiotics. Adenomyosis should be treated with danazol or GnRH agonists and not OCs.

References: 81, 83, 274

NOTES

#11 Vaginal Changes/Cervical Changes

VAGINAL CHANGES

Clinical Information
Vaginal infections that may be increased in OC users include:
- Vaginitis
- Vulvitis
- Moniliasis (yeast, fungus)
- Trichomoniasis
- HIV-1

Vaginal infections whose treatments may affect OC effectiveness include hemophilus vaginitis.

Vaginitis, vulvitis, and moniliasis have been reported to be increased in OC users in some studies. OCs do not interfere with treatment of moniliasis with miconazole nitrate cream. The incidence of trichomoniasis is unchanged or decreased by OC use.

Leukorrhea, or mucoid discharge identical to the egg white-like discharge that precedes ovulation, is sometimes noted with high-estrogenic activity OCs. This is due to the effect of estrogen on cervical and endometrial glands and is opposed by progestins.

OC users had twice the incidence of moniliasis in the Royal College of General Practitioners (RCGP) study. Moniliasis is more common during pregnancy when progesterone levels are high. Vaginitis is more common when estrogenic activity is low. Vaginitis and vulvitis may also be related to progestational or androgenic activity.

Pelvic inflammatory disease (PID) is significantly decreased in OC users. However, OCs do not offer any protection against sexually transmitted diseases (STDs), such as herpes genitalis.

HIV-1-infected cells were significantly increased in endocervical and vaginal swabs from patients who used Depo-Provera® (odds ratio [OR] = 2.9) and both low-dose (OR = 3.8) and high-dose (OR = 12.3) OCs. Vitamin A was also associated with increased vaginal HIV-1 shedding (Ref 279).

Causal Factors

Cervical hypertrophy and exstrophy often accompany a leukorrheic discharge related to excess estrogen. Microscopic examination of such discharge reveals numerous epithelial cells caused by high estrogenic activity. The opposite effect, a lack of sufficient lubrication and a dry vagina, may be due to an excessive progestational effect or a lack of estrogen.

OCs are intended to prevent pregnancy and do not protect against HIV infection, AIDs, and other sexually transmitted diseases.

-FDA Package Insert Labeling

Management

The cervix should always be examined before making a disposition.

Mucoid discharge, especially when cervical hypertrophy is also present, can be treated by switching patients to OCs with less estrogenic activities.

Persistent or recurrent vaginitis, moniliasis, or other local infections may necessitate a switch to an OC with less progestational activity.

Moniliasis may be treated by a vaginal antifungal agent such as a one-day course of tioconazole or a three- to seven-day course of terconazole (Terazol®, Ortho), miconazole nitrate (Monistat®, Ortho), econazole nitrate, or clotrimazole. A once-a-week application of one of the latter four therapies may reduce the incidence of recurrence.

Herpes genitalis is not related to OC use. No specific treatment is known. Nonoxynol and related drugs used in vaginal spermicidal products are toxic to herpes genitalis *in vitro*. Herpes may be treated with acyclovir (Zovirax®). Use of these products together with condoms should reduce the possibility of acquiring or spreading herpes genitalis.

Trichomoniasis is best treated by metronidazole, but the contraceptive effectiveness of OCs is reduced with its use; therefore, additional contraceptive measures should be used during this treatment regimen.

Hemophilis vaginalis (bacterial vaginosis) can be treated with either the oral form or the newer vaginal application of metronidazole or clindamycin.

If cervical hypertrophy or exstrophy occurs, patients should be switched to OCs with less estrogenic activities. If repeated cervicitis occurs, patients should be switched to OCs with lower progestational and androgenic activities.

References: 8, 77, 83, 141, 279, 314, 356, 473

CERVICAL CHANGES

Cervicitis

Chlamydia trachomatis endocervicitis is more common in OC users. At the same time, the incidence of symptomatic PID is decreased (Ref 264, 369, 411).

Causal Factors

Use of OCs is associated with increased cervical ectopy (endocervical cells advancing onto the ectocervix) (Ref 138). Endocervical cells are the primary site for attachment of *C. trachomatis and Neisseria gonorrhea*.

Cervical hypertrophy and exstrophy are due to the estrogen components of OCs and result from accelerated growth of endocervical cells onto the exterior of the cervix. Cervicitis is related to the progestin content.

Management

Use of newer low-dose combination and triphasic OCs may reduce the incidence of cervical ectopy.

Neoplasm

Some studies suggest that oral contraceptive use has been associated with an increase in the risk of cervical intraepithelial neoplasia in some populations of women. However, there continues to be controversy about the extent to which such findings may be due to differences in sexual behavior and other factors.

In spite of many studies of the relationship between oral contraceptive use . . . and cervical cancer, a cause and effect relationship has not been established.

-FDA Package Insert Labeling

Clinical Information

Several major studies suggest that prolonged OC use may be associated with a small increased risk of cervical neoplasm, which, apparently, is confined to women with:

- Long-term OC use
- Early sexual activity
- Multiple partners

Some epidemiological data indicate an increased risk of cervical neoplasm with OC use for 60 months or longer. The largest study, involving 46,000 women and conducted by RCGP, found no relationship between OC use and cervical neoplasia. Among studies reporting a possible relationship, one found that the overall incidence among OC users rose from 0.9 per 1,000 women per years (WYS) for those using OCs for up to two years to 2.2 per 1,000 WYS for those using OCs for eight years or more. However, the actual increase in cancer compared to nonusers was only one in 12,500 WYS.

Another study found a 68-percent increase in cervical neoplasm, but the figure did not reach clinical significance. Preliminary results from a World Health Organization (WHO) study found a relative risk (RR) of 1.2 percent in ever-users, which increased to 1.5 percent after five years of use. Another study in a developing country, which involved 24,000 women, found a higher significant association between OC use and carcinoma *in situ* (CIS) in women ages 30 to 34 who had experienced at least one pregnancy and had used OCs for 13 to 24 months. The risk for all patients, adjusted for age at first pregnancy and years of follow-up, was marginally significant. No significant differences were found for severe dysplasia.

One review of the major epidemiological studies through 1985 concluded that long-term OC use by women already at increased risk because of sexual factors appears to be associated with increased risk of cervical cancer.

A 1995 meta-analysis estimated the risk of developing cancer of the cervix from ages 20 to 54 to be 425 per 100,000 WYS in never-users. It estimated that an additional 125 cases might occur in women who used OCs for eight or more years (Ref 368). Another analysis estimated that the number of cases of cervical cancer per 100,000 U.S. women would be increased by 67 cases during their lifetimes if they used OCs for five years (Ref 62). Yet another analysis estimated that use of OCs for eight years or longer would result in 30 additional cases of cervical cancer in the U.S. (Ref 318). Another researcher estimated that, for 100,000 women who used OCs continuously from ages 16 to 35, there would be an additional 76 deaths from cervical cancer during their lifetimes (Ref 451).

There has been a greater than twofold increase in adenocarcinoma of the cervix between the early 1970s and mid-1980s in women younger than age 35. A case control study found a relative risk of 2.1 for adenocarcinoma of the cervix in users of OCs compared to nonusers (Ref 438). The risk was highest (4.4-fold) with use for longer than 12 years. No additional risk was found for age at first use. An increased risk of cervical cancer must be balanced against a 50-percent decrease in endometrial and ovarian cancers.

Cancer per se is associated with an increased hazard of developing thrombosis. The possibility of developing thrombosis might be further increased if patients with cancer use OCs.

Causal Factors

Cervical lesions associated with human papilloma virus and underlying stromal cells contain significantly more progesterone and estrogen receptors than normal cervical cells or stromal cancer (Ref 465).

The primary risk factors for cervical cancer are early sexual activity and multiple partners.

Management

Women suspected of having cancer should be evaluated without regard to OC use.

Women with proven cancer should discontinue OC use because of the increased risk of thromboembolism and the possibility of accelerated tumor growth. Other methods of birth control should be recommended for these patients.

It has been recommended that women who use OCs for more than five years should have annual Pap smears.

References: 8, 9, 18, 41, 42, 44, 83, 109, 173, 176, 212, 276, 313, 325, 330, 331, 333, 368, 424, 438

#12 Cardiovascular System

General Information
Myocardial Infarction
Cerebrovascular Accident
Pulmonary Embolism
Thrombophlebitis and Thrombosis
Other Thromboses
Hypertension

Cardiovascular Disorders

The use of oral contraceptives is associated with increased risks of several serious conditions including myocardial infarction, thromboembolism, stroke, hepatic neoplasia, and gallbladder disease, although the risk of serious morbidity and mortality increases significantly in the presence of other underlying factors such as hypertension, hyperlipidemia, hyper-cholesterolemia, obesity, and diabetes.

Practitioners prescribing oral contraceptives should be familiar with the following information relating to these risks.

The information contained in this package insert is principally based on studies carried out in patients who used oral contraceptives with formulations containing 0.05 mg or higher of estrogen. The effects of long-term use with lower dose formulations of both estrogens and progestogens remain to be determined.

Throughout this labeling, the epidemiological studies reported are of two types: retrospective or case control studies and prospective or cohort studies. Case control studies provide a measure of the relative risk of a disease. Relative risk, the ratio of the incidence of a disease among oral contraceptive users to that among non-users, cannot be assessed directly from case control studies, but the odds ratio obtained is a measure of relative risk. The relative risk does not provide information on the actual clinical occurrence of a disease. Cohort studies provide not only a measure of the relative risk but a measure of attributable risk, which is the difference in the incidence of disease between oral contraceptive users and non-users. The attributable risk does provide information about the actual occurrence of a disease in the population.

-FDA Package Insert Labeling

12

GENERAL INFORMATION

Causes of Cardiovascular Disease

Cardiovascular disease (CVD) may be due to:

- Clotting within vessels (see below):
  - Deep vein thrombosis
  - Pulmonary embolism
- Atherosclerotic changes within vessel walls (see below):
  - Hypertension

- Ischemic heart disease
- A combination of clotting and atherosclerotic effects, resulting in:
  - Myocardial infarction (MI)
  - Cerebrovascular accidents (CVA)

Clinical Information

Virtually all the excess mortality in OC users is due to CVD. Early studies involving OCs with 50 to 150 mcg mestranol found a high incidence of CVD in OC users compared to nonusers. More recent studies involving OCs with 20 to 35 mcg ethinyl estradiol (EE) and progestins with lower doses and less androgenic activities show a smaller increase and in some cases no increase in current or former OC users, except for women with specific risk factors (chiefly smoking, hypertension, and hereditary thrombophilia). The relationship of OCs to CVD has been the subject of several recent reviews (Ref 47, 347).

A 1981 Royal College of General Practitioners (RCGP) study, which gathered information on twice as many deaths as in its 1977 study, found that the relative risk (RR) of death from all vascular diseases for current OC users was increased four times and that the risk for former users was increased 4.3 times (Table 16). Most deaths in current users were due to MI, where the RR increased 6.4 times to 13 per 100,000 women per years (WYS) of use. Former users had a smaller increased risk of death due to MI (two times) but a slightly greater risk of death due to:

- Malignant hypertension
- Cerebral thrombosis
- Cerebral hemorrhage
- Pulmonary embolism

In contrast to the 1977 report, no relationship was found between the incidence of death due to CVD and the length of OC use.

Causal Factors

CVD morbidity and deaths from both venous and nonvenous causes are related to the estrogen content. OCs containing 30 mcg estrogen have lower morbidity rates than those with 50 mcg estrogen, which have lower rates than OCs containing more than 50 mcg estrogen.

Cardiovascular deaths are also related to the progestin dose and activity. Death and morbidity rates from all forms of CVD and stroke increase as the progestin dose increases from 1 to 2.5 mg norethindrone acetate and from 0.3 to 0.5 mg norgestrel, while death and morbidity rates from ischemic heart disease and venous thrombosis slightly decrease as the progestin dose increases.

One unconfirmed study found that factor VII and X levels are significantly elevated in patients using 0.15 mg desogestrel and 0.075 gestodene with 30 mcg EE but not in patients using 0.15 desogestrel with 20 mcg EE (Ref 293).

A decrease in hypertension with an increased progestin dose found in previous studies was not seen in the 1981 RCGP study. However, hypertension was found to decrease as the amount of estrogen increased.

Estrogens, especially dose levels above 50 mcg EE, induce effects in the coagulation and fibrolytic enzyme system. Nearly all studies note an increase in plasma fibrinogen concentration and factors II (prothrombin), VII, VIII, and X. These effects are questionable in OCs containing 20 mcg EE. Little difference in effects is shown between monophasic and multiphasic preparations with equal total estrogen contents.

Some 19-nor-progestins may increase the rate of atherosclerotic vascular changes by causing a decrease in plasma levels of high-density lipoprotein-(HDL) cholesterol, the cholesterol type that protects against arteriosclerotic vascular disease. Estrogen, however, increases HDL-cholesterol levels. The effect of an OC on HDL-cholesterol depends on the type of progestin and the ratio of progestin-to-estrogen (Tables 6 and 7).

Other atherosclerotic progestin-related changes include elevations of serum levels of:

- Total cholesterol
- Triglycerides
- Low-density lipoprotein (LDL)-cholesterol
- Very low-density lipoprotein (VLDL)-cholesterol

Estimates of Mortality from Contraceptive Use

One study gathered data from a variety of sources which have estimated the mortality rates associated with different methods of contraception at different ages. These estimates include the combined risk of death associated with contraceptive methods plus the risk attributable to pregnancy in the event of method failure. Each method of contraception has its specific benefits and risks. The study concluded that, with the exception of oral contraceptive users ages 35 and older who smoke and 40 and older who do not smoke, mortality associated with all methods of birth control is low and below that associated with childbirth.

-FDA Package Insert Labeling

Among OC users, the overall excess death rate annually from circulatory diseases is:

Age/Years	Annual Excess Death Rate Per 100,000 Women
15 to 34	5
34 to 44	33
45 to 49	140

The risk was concentrated among women who were:
- Older
- Long-term OC users
- Smokers

Data from several sources have been used to estimate the risk of death associated with various methods of contraception, including the combined risk of the contraceptive method itself plus the risk of pregnancy or abortion in the event of method failure (Table 2), which analyzed the risk of death:
- The mortality risk from all birth control methods is low (below that of childbirth), with the exception of OC use in smokers older than age 40
- Mortality from OC use is higher than from any other method for women older than age 40, due to increased CVD risk

The lowest mortality is associated with condom or diaphragm methods that are backed up by early abortion.

Persistence of Risk of Vascular Disease

There are three studies which have shown persistence of risk of vascular disease for ever-users of oral contraceptives. In a study in the United States, the risk of developing myocardial infarction after discontinuing oral contraceptives persists for at least nine years for women ages 40 to 49 who had used oral contraceptives for five years or more, but this increased risk was not demonstrated in other age groups. In another study in Great Britain, the risk of developing cerebrovascular disease persisted for at least six years after discontinuance of oral contraceptives, although excess risk was very small. Subarachnoid hemorrhage also has a significantly increased relative risk after termination of use of oral contraceptives. However, these studies were performed with oral contraceptive formulations containing 0.05 mg or higher of estrogen.

-FDA Package Insert Labeling

A prospective British study estimated that former users have a 2.6 times greater risk for all CVD than nonusers and that this risk remains elevated for at least six years after OCs are discontinued. A U.S. prospective study found that past OC use was associated with 5.3 times increased risk of subarachnoid hemorrhage and found some evidence that the degree of risk is related to duration of OC use.

Recent studies involving lower doses of EE and progestin show no increased risk of subarachnoid hemorrhage in former OC users.

Management

OCs should not be prescribed for women who have the following conditions:

- Ages 35 and older who smoke cigarettes
- Obesity of more than 10 percent over ideal weight
- Diabetes
- Elevated cholesterol levels
- Hypertension
- Current or past histories of thrombophlebitis
- Current hospitalization
- Immobilization of an extremity
- Family histories of CVA, MI, or pulmonary embolism before age 50
- Family histories of thrombophlebitis during pregnancy or OC use

---

Lipid Disorders
Women who are being treated for hyperlipidemias should be followed closely if they elect to use oral contraceptives. Some progestogens may elevate LDL levels and may render the control of hyperlipidemias more difficult.

-FDA Package Insert Labeling

Several large family planning programs require that women older than age 35 and those with family histories of heart attack before age 50 have annual blood cholesterol, triglyceride, and glucose determinations. Increased risk is present with elevated levels of:

- Cholesterol - 267 mg per 100 ml or higher
- Triglyceride - 207 mg per 100 ml or higher
- Fasting glucose - 105 mg per 100 ml or higher

Women with values at such ranges or higher should not take OCs.

Reducing the Risk of CVD

To reduce risks of CVD, OCs containing 35 mcg or less of estrogen and 0.5 mg or less of norethindrone or an equivalent amount of other progestins are recommended (Tables 5 and 9).

References: 24, 26, 109, 110, 187, 247, 252, 254, 255, 267, 293, 330, 331, 354, 356, 359, 404, 417, 429, 458

MYOCARDIAL INFARCTION

An increased risk of myocardial infarction has been attributed to oral contraceptive use. The risk is primarily in smokers or women with other underlying risk factors for coronary artery disease such as hypertension, hypercholesterolemia, morbid obesity, and diabetes. The relative risk of heart attack for current oral contraceptive users has been estimated to be 2 to 6. The risk is very low for women under age 30. However, there is the possibility of a risk of cardiovascular disease even in very young women who take oral contraceptives.

Oral contraceptives may compound the effects of well-known risk factors for coronary artery disease, such as hypertension, diabetes, hyperlipidemia, hypercholesterolemia, age, and obesity. In particular, some progestogens are known to decrease HDL cholesterol and impair oral glucose tolerance, while estrogens may create a state of hyperinsulinism. Oral contraceptives have been shown to increase blood pressure among users. Similar effects on risk factors have been associated with an increased risk of heart disease. Oral contraceptives must be used with caution in women with cardiovascular disease risk factors.

-FDA Package Insert Labeling

Clinical Information

From 1984 to 1992 (the last year of analysis), there was a steady decrease in deaths from MI in the U.K. from 2.1 to 1.1 per 100,000 women ages 15 to 29 and from 31.3 to 20.2 per 100,000 women ages 30 to 44. During the same period, there was an increase in deaths from venous thromboembolism (VTE) from 1.6 to 3.8 per 100,000 women ages 15 to 29 but a decrease from 7.3 to 5.4 per 100,000 women ages 30 to 54 (Ref 425). A corresponding decrease in MI occurred in men, without an increase in VTE.

An increased risk of MI has been reported in OC users, which current research shows is limited to use of first- and second-generation progestins when used in combination OCs (Ref 235). Studies in the U.K. found that the greater the number of underlying risk factors, the higher the risk of MI among users as well as nonusers of OCs.

The RR of acute MI is related to numerous factors besides use of OCs. The RR according to underlying risk factor has been estimated as (Ref 235):

- Cigarette smoking - 9.7 times
- Hypertension - 3.3 times
- High cholesterol (Type II hyperlipidemia) - 4.2 times
- Obesity (BMI):
  - BMI less than 20 - 1.0 times
  - BMI 20 to 24 - 1.7 times
  - BMI 25 to 29 - 3.7 times*
  - BMI greater than 29 - 4.8 times
- Diabetes - 2.5 times
- History of pre-eclamptic toxemia
- Family history of MI - 3.7 times
- Parity - 2.8 times

*BMI of 25 is equal to a weight of 145 for a height of 5'4"

The greater the number of underlying risk factors, the higher the risk of MI among OC users as well as nonusers:

- One factor increased the risk four times
- Two factors increased the risk 10 times
- Three factors increased the risk 78 times

Women with blood type O may be at less risk than those with type A, B, or AB.

In determining the importance of these RRs, the baseline rates for various age groups must be given serious consideration. The importance of other predisposing conditions in determining relative and absolute risks has not yet been quantified. It is likely that some synergistic action exists but perhaps to a lesser extent.

In a transnational study, the odds ratio (OR) for MI was 1.07 when blood pressure was checked before prescribing OCs compared to 2.76 when blood pressure was not checked before OCs were prescribed (Ref 235).

Causal Factors
Effects of Cigarette Smoking

Cigarette Smoking

Cigarette smoking increases the risk of serious cardiovascular side effects from oral contraceptive use. This risk increases with age and with heavy smoking (15 or more cigarettes per day) and is quite marked in women over 35 years of age. Women who use oral contraceptives should be strongly advised not to smoke.

Smoking in combination with oral contraceptive use has been shown to contribute substantially to the incidence of myocardial infarction in women 35 or older, with smoking accounting for the majority of excess cases.

Mortality rates associated with circulatory disease have been shown to increase substantially in smokers over the age of 35 and non-smokers over the age of 40 among women who use oral contraceptives.

-FDA Package Insert Labeling

It is now well-recognized that the risk of MI in OC users is almost entirely confined to those who are older than age 35 and who also smoke (Table 17). No deaths from MI associated with OC use have been reported in nonsmokers younger than age 25. The excess risk from OC use in nonsmokers vs smokers, rated by age, is:

Age/Years	Mortality	
	Nonsmokers	**Smokers**
25 to 34	1 per 59,000	1 per 10,000
35 to 44	1 per 6,600	1 per 2,100
Over 45	1 per 2,500	1 per 500

The effect of smoking on MI was greatest for first-generation progestins and least for third-generation progestins when used in combination OCs (Ref 235):
- First-generation progestin OCs OR = 19.5
- Second-generation progestin OCs OR = 9.5
- Third-generation progestin OCs OR = 3.8

In the same study, there was no increased risk to OC users who were former smokers.

There is a demonstrated relationship between the number of cigarettes smoked per day and the risk of fatal or nonfatal MI:

Cigarettes Per Day	Times MI Risk Is Increased
Less than 15	1.2 times
15 to 24	4.1 times
More than 24	11.3 times

Decreased fibrinolytic activity in vessel walls was demonstrated in both women who used OCs for more than five years and in women who smoked more than 10 cigarettes per day, suggesting the possibility of a synergistic effect (Ref 213).

It is the considered opinion of many knowledgeable experts that women ages 35 and older who smoke cigarettes should not use OCs.

Progestin Type

The risk of developing MI while taking OCs is decreased by 73 percent in users of third-generation progestin OCs compared to users of second-generation progestin OCs. A transnational European study of MI found that, when controlled for duration of use and cigarette smoking, the RR of MI with third-generation OCs containing desogestrel or gestodene compared to nonuse was close to 1.0. For second-generation OCs, relative to nonuse, the RR was 3.1; and for third-generation compared to second-generation OCs, the RR was 0.31 (Ref 236).

In an updated report, based on a larger sample, the RR for third-generation progestins compared to nonuse was 0.8, for second-generation progestins compared to nonuse was 2.8, and for third-generation compared to second-generation was 0.27 and significant (95 percent confidence interval [CI] 0.1 to 1.0) (Ref 233).

This illustrates the decrease with time and increased sample size that occurs in most OC morbidity studies. Another study based on the U.K. General Practice Database found no significant difference between second- and third-generation progestins (Ref 194). A. U.S. health maintenance organization (HMO)-based study found an adjusted (for smoking and age) OR of 1.14 for mostly sub-50 mcg (90 percent) OC users vs nonusers (Ref 383). In this study, most patients were free of risk factors, e.g., patients with hypertension were not prescribed OCs. The OR for former OC users compared to nonusers was 0.6 in the same study.

Other studies that have compared sub-50 mcg EE to 50 mcg EE OCs, irrespective of progestin type, have found the RR of developing MI compared to nonusers to be 2.2 for sub-50 mcg vs 3.1 to 4.2 for 50 mcg OCs (Ref 2).

Management

MI can be prevented by use of sub-50 mcg EE OCs, especially if they contain third-generation progestins, and by not prescribing OCs for patients with additional risk factors, particularly smoking, hypertension, family history of MI, and obesity.

Clinicians who prescribe OCs should be aware of the possibility of MI in all patients, not just OC users, and should be prepared to respond promptly to patients who report symptoms of possible MI. Mortality and morbidity can be substantially reduced if treatment with thrombolytic agents is initiated within three hours (Ref 431).

Also see *Management* under *General Information*, above.

References: 2, 26, 47, 109, 110, 139, 141, 186, 187, 190, 192, 213, 223, 235, 252, 253, 254, 255, 267, 293, 330, 347, 425, 469, 502

An increase in both the relative and attributable risks of cerebrovascular events (thrombotic and hemorrhagic strokes) has been shown in users of oral contraceptives. In general, the risk is greatest among older (> 35 years), hypertensive women who also smoke. Hypertension was found to be a risk factor for both users and non-users for both types of strokes, while smoking interacted to increase the risk for hemorrhagic strokes.

In a large study, the relative risk of thrombotic strokes has been shown to range from 3 for normotensive users to 14 for users with severe hypertension. The relative risk of hemorrhagic stroke is reported to be 1.2 for non-smokers who used oral contraceptives, 2.6 for smokers who did not use oral contraceptives, 7.6 for smokers who used oral contraceptives, 1.8 for normotensive users and 25.7 for users with severe hypertension. The attributable risk also is greater in women 35 and older and among smokers.

-FDA Package Insert Labeling

Clinical Information

CVA includes:

- Stroke
- Cerebral thrombosis
- Cerebral hemorrhage
- Subarachnoid hemorrhage

In early studies involving 50 to 150 mcg estrogen OCs, CVAs of all types occurred in 41 per 100,000 women years (WYS) compared to 10 per 100,000 WYS for nonusers.

Other factors significantly increase the risk of stroke. A 1995 Danish study of women ages 15 to 44 who had thrombotic strokes found the OR, adjusted by multivariate analysis, to be 5.4 for diabetes, 3.1 for hypertension, 2.8 for migraine, and 5.3 for previous noncerebral vascular thrombosis (Ref 239). The increased risk for stroke in patients with these factors was the same in OC users and nonusers.

In a 1975 collaborative U.S. study of cerebrovascular disorders in women with and without predisposing causes, the estimated risk of hemorrhagic stroke was two times greater in OC users than nonusers and the risk of thrombotic stroke was four to 9.5 times greater.

In a later RCGP study still involving users of 50 to 100 mcg estrogen OCs, deaths from subarachnoid hemorrhage were increased three times (to 7.3 per 100,000 WYS) in OC users compared to controls; no increase was shown in deaths due to:

- Cerebral thrombosis
- Hemorrhage
- Embolism

After OCs were discontinued, the risk of subarachnoid hemorrhage remained high, and the risk of thrombosis and/or embolism was three times that of women who never used OCs.

There is no increased risk of stroke in patients who use sub-50 mcg EE OCs and do not smoke. In a study that suggested a strong relationship between hypertension and smoking, OC use was found to be only weakly related to the risk of subarachnoid hemorrhage. For nonhemorrhagic stroke, OC use was a clear risk factor but was confined to current OC users; hypertension and smoking had little effect. In the same study, no strokes were observed among women using OCs containing less than 50 mcg estrogen.

In a study of all women in Denmark (ages 15 to 44) who experienced CVAs during 1985 to 1989, the OR for cerebral thrombotic attack was (Ref 238):

- 2.9 percent for those taking 50 mcg estrogen OCs
- 1.8 percent for those taking 30 to 40 mcg estrogen OCs
- 0.9 percent for those taking progestin-only pills

These ratios did not change with age or years of use. Cigarette smoking increased the risk of CVA by 50 percent independently of OCs in this study.

A 1996 case control study found the adjusted OR for cerebral ischemic infarction among current users of sub-50 mcg EE OCs compared to nonusers was 0.65 and for hemorrhagic stroke was 1.02 (Ref 319). The overall incidence of ischemic and hemorrhagic stroke in this population was 5.4 and 5.6 per 100,000 WYS, respectively. The adjusted OR for former users of sub-50 mcg OCs compared to never users was 1.0 for both ischemic and hemorrhagic stroke. The crude incidence of ischemic stroke was increased for women who smoked, had hypertension or diabetes, were obese, or were African-American; and the incidence of hemorrhagic stroke was increased for women with all these factors except obesity in the same study (Ref 319). There was a positive correlation between smoking and current OC use for hemorrhagic stroke (OR = 3.6) but not for ischemic stroke. In three other case control studies, the OR for hemorrhagic stroke in users of sub-50 mcg OCs were also low: 1.1 (Ref 427), 1.5 (Ref 160), and 0.89 (Ref 245).

In a 1996 World Health Organization (WHO) Study, the RR of ischemic stroke was 1.53 (not significant) in women who used sub-50 mcg OCs, and there was no increase in hemorrhagic stroke (Ref 487, 488). The same study estimated the annual attributable risk to be two per 100,000 WYS in those using sub-50 mcg OCs.

Data from the 1991 RCGP study found the adjusted OR for thrombotic stroke was 0.6 in women who used sub-50 mcg OCs and did not smoke (Ref 160). The Oxford Family Planning study of 17,000 OC users recorded no cases of thrombotic stroke in women who used sub-50 mcg OCs compared to 13 cases in women who used OCs with 50 mcg estrogen or higher (Ref 452).

Causal Factors

Thrombotic stroke is not significantly affected by progestin type. In a 1997 case control hospital study, the OR, adjusted for age, smoking, hypertension, obesity, family history, and duration of OC use, was 4.4 for first-generation progestin OCs, 3.4 for second-generation progestin OCs, and 3.9 for third-generation progestin OCs. The OR for all preparations was lower if blood pressure was checked before OC prescription (Ref 166).

An older report found that women who experienced cerebrovascular insufficiency while using OCs were more likely to have mitral valve prolapse. Other reports have found mitral valve prolapse in 40 percent of patients younger than age 45 with cerebral ischemia compared to six to eight percent of controls.

CVAs are often preceded by persistent headache for weeks or months and/or by transient hemiparesis. CVAs are rarely precipitated by mild hypertension but may be caused by extreme hypertension.

See *Causal Factors* under *General Information*, above, for additional factors.

Management

Women with migraines that worsen while taking OCs should discontinue OC use, even though their conditions may improve with use of OCs containing 30 mcg or less of estrogen. Women who develop persistent headaches and/or transient hemiparesis while taking OCs should discontinue use immediately. Women with family histories of CVAs or stroke in close relatives or with personal histories of transient hemiparesis may be at increased risk of experiencing the same conditions if they take OCs.

Thrombotic stroke during OC use may be prevented by use of sub-50 mcg estrogen preparations.

Clinicians who prescribe OCs should be aware of the possibility of thrombotic stroke in all patients, not just OC users, and should be prepared to respond promptly to patients who report symptoms or have evidence of stroke. Mortality and morbidity can be substantially reduced if treatment with thrombolytic agents is initiated within three hours (Ref 284).

References: 26, 63, 64, 109, 110, 160, 166, 186, 187, 238, 239, 245, 316, 319, 330, 331, 354, 356, 427, 452, 457, 459, 487, 488

PULMONARY EMBOLISM

Clinical Information

In the 1960s, the excess mortality rate due to pulmonary embolism or stroke was one to 3.5 deaths annually per 100,000 OC users (Table 16). Pulmonary embolism is now rare due to use of sub 50 mcg estrogen OCs.

Pulmonary embolism is characterized by:
• Shortness of breath

- Chest pain
- Hemoptysis (coughing of blood)

Not all these symptoms need exist at once. The pain may be mild or may be referred elsewhere (to the shoulder or upper abdomen).

Other, more benign conditions may mimic the symptoms of pulmonary embolism, including:
- Pleurisy
- Spontaneous rupture of the lung
- Trauma to rib or cartilage
- Pneumonia

Most patients survive if treatment is started early.

Causal Factors

See *Causal Factors*, below, under *Thrombophlebitis and Thrombosis* and *Causes of Cardiovascular Disease* under *General Information,* above.

Management

When pulmonary embolism is suspected because of any of the symptoms listed above, immediate steps to establish a diagnosis must be taken, including chest x-rays and radiographic lung scans, if available.

Once the diagnosis is established, immediate anticoagulant therapy is necessary. Ligation of the vena cava may be required if repeated embolism occurs.

References: 26, 186, 187, 355, 356, 359, 365, 454, 459

THROMBOPHLEBITIS AND THROMBOSIS

Thromboembolism

An increased risk of thromboembolic and thrombotic disease associated with the use of oral contraceptives is well established. Case control studies have found the relative risk of users compared to non-users to be three for the first episode of superficial venous thrombosis, four to 11 for deep vein thrombosis or pulmonary embolism, and 1.5 to 6 for women with predisposing conditions for venous thromboembolic disease. One cohort study has shown the relative risk to be somewhat lower, about three for new cases (subjects with no past history of venous thrombosis or varicose veins), and about 4.5 for new cases requiring hospitalization. The risk of thromboembolic disease due to oral contraceptives is not related to length of use and disappears after pill use is stopped.

-FDA Package Insert Labeling

Clinical Information

Signs of superficial and deep vein thrombosis include:

- Pain to the touch, localized to an extremity
- Swelling
- Warmth
- Altered blood flow (detected by ultrasonography or dye injection)

An increased risk of thrombotic disease was associated with use of OCs containing 75 mcg or more EE. Numerous British and U.S. studies have demonstrated an increased risk of fatal and nonfatal VTE, estimating that OC users are four to 11 times more likely to develop these diseases without evident cause. Superficial thrombosis of the leg was increased by 50 percent from a rate of two per 1,000 WYS to three per 1,000 WYS. Deep vein thrombosis was increased four-to-seven fold, to a rate of 0.5 per 1,000 WYS of OC use.

In 1995 and 1996, four studies (Ref 32, 193, 486, 489) found that deep venous thrombosis and pulmonary embolism occurred approximately twice as often in users of OCs containing greater than 50 mcg EE and desogestrel (DS) or gestodene (GS) as in OCs containing norgestrel (NG) or levonorgestrel (LNG). However, these studies did not control for length of use (venous thrombosis is more likely to occur in first year of OC use), age, smoking, or weight (10 percent more women prescribed DS were overweight). When these factors were controlled, the ORs were 3.2 (95 percent, 2.3 to 4.3) for combination OCs containing NG and LNG vs no use and 4.8 (45 percent, 3.4 to 6.7) for combination OCs containing DS and GS vs no use. Any increase in thrombosis must be balanced against an approximately three times higher risk of MI in users of NG and LNG combination OCs compared to DS and GS (Ref 236). The differences between NG/LNG and DS/GS were not significant (Ref 396).

The highest rate of VTE with any OC occurs during the first years after its introduction (Ref 338, 395). Thus, the incidence of VTE decreased from 12 to 13 per 10,000

WYS in the early 1970s (when many women were using OCs with more than 50 mcg estrogen and first-generation progestins) to seven to 11 per 10,000 WYS during the 1980s for 50 mcg estrogen and finally to four per 10,000 WYS for 30 to 35 mcg EE) (Ref 395).

A similar decrease occurred for second-generation progestins from 3.9 to 4.2 in 1988 to 1.0 to 1.6 in 1996, although the dose of estrogen (30 to 35 mcg EE) did not change (Ref 395).

Initial rates of VTE for third-generation progestins were similar to initial rates for second-generation progestins in 1988. Later studies found the rate of VTE to be 2.1 per 10,000 WYS, not significantly different from second-generation progestins after adjustment for length of use, first-time starters, and additional risk factors. By comparison, absolute rates for VTE as high as 10 per 10,000 WYS have been reported for nonusers (Ref 273).

In a transnational study, the OR of third- vs second-generation progestins decreased with time, from 2.7 in 1993 to 1.6 in 1994 and 1.2 in 1995 (Ref 395). In a smaller study, the OR of third- vs second-generation progestins decreased from 2.7 in 1991 to 1992 to 2.0 in 1993 to 1994 (Ref 193). In a study in which cases and controls were exactly matched for age, the OR for VTE in third- vs second-generation progestins was 0.8 (Ref 395).

The OR for VTE for triphasic levonorgestrel (LNG) vs monophasic LNG with the same EE content was 2.1 shortly after the introduction of triphasic LNG, and the OR for VTE for desogestrel (DG) with 30 mcg EE vs monophasic LNG was higher (2.5) than the OR for DG with 30 mcg EE vs monophasic LNG (1.2).

In a case control study (Ref 106), this introductory effect has been explained by the tendency of clinicians to prescribe the newest OCs, which frequently have lower doses of estrogen and progestin, for their older or higher-risk patients. Any possible increase in the incidence of VTE in third- vs second-generation progestins must be balanced against the decreased incidence of MI for third- (OR = 0.28) vs second-generation progestins (Ref 485) and against the low incidence of fatality in VTE, estimated to be 1.5 to 3.0 per one million second- and third-generation progestin OC users compared to a background incidence of fatality from VTE of six per one million women ages 15 to 44 (Ref 201).

Fatal cases of VTE are frequently preceded by symptoms of lesser involvement. Most cases of thromboembolism do not end fatally.

Causal Factors

Hypercoagulability, due to estrogen, increases the possibility of a clot forming in an obstructed or dilated vein.

Thrombophlebitis and deep vein thrombosis are caused by the dilation of veins, which results in a slowing of the rate of blood flow. The dilation of smooth muscle structures (including vein walls), caused by progesterone, is common during pregnancy and occurs in some OC users. Other smooth muscle structures that may dilate under the influence of progestins include veins, ureters, bile ducts, and bowels.

Most thrombophlebitis and deep vein thrombosis cases are associated with factors other than OC use, including:

- Obesity
- Major surgery
- Injury or immobilization of an extremity
- Inherited plasma protein abnormalities (thrombophilias)

Thrombophilias

Thrombophilias include:

- Protein C deficiency
- Protein S deficiency
- Antithrombin III deficiency, inherited as autosomal dominant traits
- Leiden factor V mutation

Protein C is a vitamin K-dependent anticoagulant plasma protein. It is activated as thrombin binds to the endothelial surface receptor thrombomodulin. Protein

S functions as a co-factor in this pathway. Activated protein C (APC) prevents clot formation at the surface of endothelium or platelets by inhibiting the effect of factor V or VIII in the clotting cascade. Leiden factor V mutation involves APC resistance. It is present in five percent of the general population and up to 40 percent of patients with histories of VTE (Ref 412). The prevalence of protein C and S in the general population is 0.5 percent, rising to four percent in patients with histories of VTE (Ref 4). Patients with thrombophilias, especially Leiden factor V mutation, causes an eightfold increase in VTE. This rises to 30-fold if they use OCs, but the actual incidence remains low (28.5 per 10,000 WYS of use) (Ref 444).

One study suggested that one of the third-generation progestins, gestodene, might retard the inactivation and elimination of EE (Ref 201). This could not be confirmed by other studies (Ref 159, 302). An as-yet unconfirmed study found that women who used third-generation progestins acquired a degree of resistance to the protein C anticoagulant system similar to the APC resistance seen in persons with Leiden factor V mutation, whereas women using second-generation progestins showed only about half this effect (Ref 350). Other studies have disputed this finding (Ref 395).

See *Cardiovascular Disease*, *Causal Factors*, above, for additional information.

Management

OCs should be discontinued and other birth control methods used if VTE is suspected. A diagnosis should be established by clinical and radiological methods.

Superficial thrombophlebitis may be treated by:
- Bed rest
- Heat
- Elevation of the extremity
- Anti-inflammatory agents (optional)

Deep vein thrombosis must be treated by anticoagulant therapy.

Baseline lung x-rays should be taken and close observation of patients with deep vein thrombosis is necessary to detect symptoms of pulmonary embolism.

OCs should not be restarted in patients who have experienced deep vein thrombosis.

The low incidence of Leiden factor V mutation (five percent) and other thrombophilias in the general population and the low risk of VTE in women with Leiden factor V mutation who use OCs (less than 30 per 10,000 WYS) make screening of all patients impractical. Nevertheless, screening may be indicated in women with personal or family histories of thrombosis.

Pre- and Postoperative Thromboembolism

> A two- to sixfold increase in relative risk of post-operative thromboembolic complications has been reported with the use of oral contraceptives. If feasible, oral contraceptives should be discontinued at least four weeks prior to and for two weeks after elective surgery and during and following prolonged immobilization. Since the immediate postpartum period also is associated with an increased risk of thromboembolism, oral contraceptives should be started no earlier than four to six weeks after delivery in women who elect not to breastfeed.
>
> -FDA Package Insert Labeling

Combination OCs should be discontinued four weeks before elective surgery and not restarted until two weeks postsurgery. Combination OCs should not be started until four to six weeks postpartum. Other contraceptive methods should be recommended during these times.

References: 4, 32, 35, 106, 109, 110, 150, 159, 186, 187, 193, 201, 236, 251, 273, 284, 302, 330, 331, 350, 355, 356, 357, 365, 395, 396, 412, 431, 439, 444, 450, 453, 454, 469, 485, 486, 489

OTHER THROMBOSES

Mesenteric Artery or Vein Thrombosis

Arterial thrombosis is only half as common as mesenteric vein thrombosis but is twice as likely to cause death. In a review of 21 OC-related cases, the mortality was 50 percent. Abdominal pain was present in all patients for two or more weeks, due to small bowel ischemia.

In addition to persistent abdominal pain, other symptoms may include:

- Fever
- Elevated white blood cell count
- Vomiting
- Diarrhea
- Bloody stools or hematemesis (depending on the location in the bowel)

An upper gastrointestinal (GI) series, with follow-through, will show a narrowing of a small bowel segment.

References: 19, 182, 232, 294, 442, 476

Splenic Artery Thrombosis

Only one case of splenic artery thrombosis in an OC user has been reported. The patient presented with upper left-quadrant pain of two weeks' duration and leukocytosis of 14,000 (Ref 476).

An uneventful recovery followed the patient's splenectomy.

Inferior Vena Cava Thrombosis

A case of thrombosis of the entire inferior vena cava and renal, pelvic, and femoral veins has been reported. The 24-year-old patient presented with a backache of 10 days' duration and swelling of the lower extremities (Ref 19).

The diagnosis was made by computed tomography. The patient was successfully treated with heparin.

Hepatic Vein Thrombosis

At least 47 cases of hepatic vein thrombosis (Budd-Chiari syndrome) have been reported in OC users (Ref 232). Survival was 50 percent in both surgically and medically treated patients and was related to early diagnosis and treatment. The relative risk for OC users has been calculated as 2.4 compared to nonusers (Ref 442).

Symptoms are pain and abdominal swelling. Elevated alkaline phosphatase may be the only abnormal lab value.

HYPERTENSION

Elevated Blood Pressure
An increase in blood pressure has been reported in women taking oral contraceptives. The incidence of risk also was reported to increase with continued use and among older women. Data from the Royal College of General Practitioners and subsequent randomized trials have shown that the incidence of hypertension increases with increasing concentrations of progestogens.

-FDA Package Insert Labeling

Clinical Information

Women who used OCs were six times more likely to develop hypertension than nonusers in early studies. OC-related hypertension, when it occurs, is usually mild to moderate (10 to 20 mm Hg diastolic and 20 to 40 mm Hg systolic), and the hypertension is usually reversible within one to three months after OCs are discontinued. A few cases progressing to malignant hypertension have been reported.

The probability of developing hypertension increases with age and duration of OC use, though hypertension may appear at any time during OC use and is not limited to the first months of use. Hypertension will appear in five percent of those who take OCs for five years.

In a regression analysis of blood pressure changes over time, the average increase in systolic pressure was 4.1 mm Hg soon after beginning OCs and was reversed soon after discontinuance. The average diastolic effect after beginning OCs was an insignificant increase of 1 mm Hg, but diastolic pressure levels increased with duration of use (0.5 mm Hg per year, $p = 0.0009$).

Women with family histories of hypertension or toxemia in pregnancy are more likely to develop hypertension while using OCs. In such cases, the OC is believed to unmask an underlying prehypertensive condition.

No deaths from malignant hypertension among current users were reported in the most recent RCGP study.

Causal Factors

Hypertension in OC users appears to be associated with the progestin component. Elevated blood pressure has not been found in women taking estrogen for menopausal hormone replacement.

The effect of progestins on blood pressure is related to the dose and potency and may be synergistic with estrogen (see Section #3). In one study, both levonorgestrel (LNG) 0.15 mg and ethynodiol diacetate 2 mg raised systolic and diastolic pressures significantly, while lower doses of the same progestins (0.075 and 0.5 mg, respectively) had no effect.

See also *Causes of Cardiovascular Disease* and *Causal Factors*, above.

Management

Women with histories of hypertension or hypertension-related diseases or renal disease should be encouraged to use another method of contraception. If women elect to use oral contraceptives, they should be monitored closely and, if significant elevation of blood pressure occurs, oral contraceptives should be discontinued. For most women, elevated blood pressure will return to normal after stopping oral contraceptives and there is no difference in the occurrence of hypertension among ever- and never-users.

-FDA Package Insert Labeling

Mild increases in blood pressure may be treated initially by switching patients to OCs with less progestin activities and, if possible, the same estrogen contents. Patients should allow three months for return to normal blood pressures to occur. If hypertension continues, OCs should be stopped and alternative contraceptive methods considered.

Antihypertensive medications should not be used along with OCs because of the differing mechanisms of actions of the two drug types. Stopping either the medication or the OC might result in an unpredictable change in blood pressure.

References: 26, 34, 69, 82, 109, 110, 113, 208, 225, 256, 316, 330, 331, 356, 358, 359, 393, 459

#13 Endocrine/Metabolic Systems

Diabetes Mellitus
Adrenal Changes
Thyroid Changes

DIABETES MELLITUS

Oral contraceptives have been shown to impair oral glucose tolerance. Oral contraceptives containing greater than 0.075 mg of estrogen cause glucose intolerance with impaired insulin secretion, while lower doses of estrogen may produce less glucose intolerance. Progestogens increase insulin secretion and create insulin resistance, this effect varying with different progestational agents. However, in the non-diabetic woman, oral contraceptives appear to have no effect on fasting blood glucose. Because of these demonstrated effects, prediabetic and diabetic women should be carefully observed while taking oral contraceptives.

Some women may develop persistent hypertriglyceridemia while on the pill. Changes in serum triglyceride and lipoprotein levels have been reported in oral contraceptive users.

-FDA Package Insert Labeling

Clinical Information

The incidence of diabetes mellitus (DM) is approximately:

- Six percent in Caucasian Americans
- 10 percent in African-Americans
- 14 percent in Mexican-Americans

More than 90 percent of the diabetic population has noninsulin-dependent diabetes (NIDDM), or Type II diabetes, and 80 percent of these people are overweight. Approximately half of patients with NIDDM have no symptoms. Insulin-dependent diabetes (IDDM), or Type I diabetes, accounts for 10 percent of the total. Not included in these figures are gestational diabetes and impaired glucose tolerance (IGT). Overt diabetes will develop in later life in 70 percent of women who have experienced gestational diabetes; and cardiovascular disease, hypertension, retinopathy, and/or nephropathy will eventually develop in 50 percent of these patients. IGT without overt diabetes affects eight to 10 percent of women between the ages of 20 to 40.

13.

Patients with IGT frequently have other cardiovascular risk factors, including insulin resistance, hypertension, hyperinsulinism, and hyperlipidemia. IGT with these additional symptoms is also known as syndrome X.

The diagnosis of IDDM can be made from a fasting or random (at least three hours postprandial) plasma glucose test. Confirmed levels of 140 mg/dL or greater indicate DM. Random levels of 100 mg/dL or greater indicate the need for a glucose tolerance test (GTT). If a plasma glucose of 200 mg/dL or greater is obtained two hours following a 75 gm glucose load, DM is diagnosed. Insulin resistance is indicated by a fasting glucose-to-insulin ratio of less than 5.0 (Ref 269).

Glucose tolerance changes are reversible in most patients after they discontinue OC use, but some cases of glucose intolerance that progress to insulin dependence have been reported.

Patients who require insulin prior to OC use have not been reported to experience worsening of their conditions or increased needs for insulin while taking OCs, though, theoretically, these could occur. No evidence of the development of a state of insulin resistance has been found.

Patients who develop gestational diabetes (Class A) during pregnancy and those with strong family histories of diabetes in parents or siblings have the greatest potential for having altered GTTs during OC use.

Symptoms of hypoglycemia (weakness and irritability two to four hours after a high-glucose meal) occur in some OC users, are related to progestin type and dose, and are common in women who take danazol for the treatment of endometriosis.

Causal Factors

The effects of OCs on glucose tolerance and insulin metabolism may have both short- and long-term effects on the cardiovascular system. Elevated blood sugar (hyperglycemia) increases the risk of developing coronary artery disease. In a study of 18,000 men, the incidence of coronary artery disease was doubled when the glucose level was above the 95th percentile (blood sugar greater than 96 mg/dL) two hours after a 50 gram oral glucose load. Hyperinsulinemia may derange lipid metabolism and thereby increase the risk of atherosclerotic heart disease (ASHD).

Diabetic patients requiring insulin are already predisposed to develop thromboembolic disease and heart attack. OC use by diabetic patients may further increase these risks. The relative risk (RR) of pregnancy vs the risks associated with OCs must be carefully weighed for these patients.

A review of older literature found no difference in the frequency of IDDM or NIDDM in ever-users compared to nonusers of high-dose OCs (Ref 131). Other studies had reported as much as a twofold increase in IGT in OC users. A study of low-dose OCs found that 15.4 percent of OC users had deterioration of GTTs compared to 6.3 percent of nonusers (Ref 361). Another study found that OCs that contained norethindrone (NE) did not affect insulin resistance, while low-dose combination OCs with other progestins but the same estrogen content all affected insulin resistance (Ref 136).

A decrease in glucose tolerance has been observed in a significant percentage of OC users. For this reason, prediabetic and diabetic patients should be carefully observed during OC use.

The effects of combination OCs on carbohydrate (CHO) metabolism are complex. Utilization of glucose usually deteriorates with a compensatory increase in insulin secretion during OC use. Progestins cause a decrease and estrogens an increase in the number of insulin receptors on the cell membrane.

Estrogens may slow the uptake of glucose from the gastrointestinal (GI) tract. High-estrogen OCs cause the greatest elevation in the glucose tolerance curve (GTC) and a delay in the peak.

During a GTT, insulin levels are elevated in all OC users except those taking pregnane-derived progestins (medroxyprogesterone acetate [MPA], megestrol). In particular, the early insulin response to glucose is exaggerated, but the hyperinsulinemia continues and may be found even in a fasting state. Changes in insulin levels occur in users of OCs that contain:

- Norgestrel, levonorgestrel - Greatest elevation
- Ethynodiol diacetate - Intermediate elevation
- Desogestrel, gestodene, norethindrone, norethindrone acetate and norgestimate - Least elevation

Investigations carried on for two years or longer show that the deterioration in the GTC is progressive and is accompanied by a persistent elevation of insulin levels in relation to the serum glucose level (hyperinsulinemia). Although the GTC deteriorates progressively with time, the insulin level does not increase further after its initial rise. This may indicate that the effect of the progestin reaches a maximum early and does not increase further.

A significant deterioration in the GTT and hyperinsulinemia also occurs in women taking triphasic OCs and OCs containing 0.15 LNG plus 30 mcg ethinyl estradiol (EE). Hyperinsulinemia does not seem to occur in women taking low-dose OCs containing 0.4 or 0.5 mg norethindrone combined with 35 mcg EE or triphasic OCs containing norethindrone.

A study by Shoupe and Kjos (Ref 379) of the effects of low-dose OCs on obese patients with histories of Class A1 or Class A2 gestational diabetes confirms this. The initial data suggest that low-dose monophasic norethindrone OCs do not affect glucose tolerance significantly at three, six, and 13 months as occurred in the control group and patients taking levonorgestrel and that their effects are significantly less than those of triphasic OCs.

A Royal College of General Practitioners (RCGP) study found a 6.9-fold greater risk of MI in diabetic patients taking low-dose OCs compared to controls (Ref 73). However, a Copenhagen study found only a 1.8-fold increased risk under the same conditions (Ref 192).

In one study of women with histories of gestational diabetes, low-dose combination norethindrone and norethindrone acetate OCs resulted in minimal GTT changes (Ref 379). Another study found no changes in GTTs in triphasic OC users (Ref 386). After six months' use of combination OCs containing levonorgestrel, 27 percent of former gestational diabetes patients developed abnormal GTTs (Ref 224). Carbohydrate metabolism appears to be less affected by the new progestins desogestrel, gestodene, and norgestimate than by older, second-generation progestins (Ref 394). Progestin implants have not been shown to alter glucose levels in healthy women and only a slight increase in fasting glucose levels in one study. In patients with IDDM who used high- and low-dose first-generation and triphasic second-generation OCs, there were no changes in fasting glucose levels or 24-hour insulin requirements or serum cholesterol changes (Ref 385).

Management

Pregnancy may aggravate complications of DM, such as retinopathy, nephropathy, and coronary artery disease. A pregnant woman with IDDM is more likely to experience complications, such as hypertension and urinary tract infection, and her fetus is at increased risk for congenital malformations, prematurity, stillbirth, neonatal morbidity, and diabetes in later life (Ref 269). For this reason, all pregnancies in diabetic women should be planned. Women with IDDM need the most effective contraception available. The benefits of OCs, implants, and injectable progestins clearly outweigh the risks of these agents. In selecting OCs, low-dose monophasics or triphasics that limit the amount or degree of androgenic activity of the progestin are the best choices for women with IDDM or histories of gestational diabetes. Table 9 lists OCs that fit this description (Groups 2 and 4-8). The fact that an OC is low-dose or multiphasic does not guarantee that it has low androgen activity. Additionally, patients with IGT or who have insulin-resistance should concentrate on weight loss.

Women at high risk for diabetes should initially be given OCs with progestin activities equal to or less than 0.5 mg norethindrone.

Prior to starting OCs and annually during OC use, patients at risk for DM should have fasting blood sugar (FBS) determinations.

Patients who have family histories of diabetes in grandparents, parents, or siblings and patients who have had gestational diabetes should have two-hour postprandial sugar tests as a minimum, though full GTTs are preferable for these patients before they start OCs. These tests should be repeated during the second or third cycle of OC use. If a marked change is observed in glucose tolerance (significantly higher serum glucose levels), these patients should stop OC use. Once their glucose levels return to normal, these patients may be switched to OCs with lower estrogen/progesterone activities and the pills restarted. If their glucose levels again become abnormal, patients should permanently discontinue OC use and use alternative contraceptive methods. Oral hypoglycemic medications should not be used in order that OCs may be continued.

Diabetic OC users are at increased risk of cardiovascular disease (CVD). Clinicians may wish to counsel these patients who have achieved their desired family size about permanent contraception (sterilization).

Patients experiencing symptoms of hypoglycemia (feeling faint or nervous three to four hours after eating) should be switched to OCs with lower progestational and androgenic or greater estrogenic activities. Low-carbohydrate/high-protein diet modification should also be prescribed.

References: 22, 78, 83, 88, 93, 109, 110, 125, 131, 136, 192, 203, 224, 247, 256, 269, 361, 378, 379, 385, 386, 394, 418, 497, 499, 501, 502

ADRENAL CHANGES

Clinical Information

Adrenal changes during OC use involve a slight rise in free cortisol levels, which may be clinically significant, and increases in protein-bound serum cortisol levels.

Progesterone and progestins derived from progesterone are bound to corticosteroid binding globulin (CSBG) but not to sex steroid binding globulin (SSBG); those derived from 19-nor-testosterone are not bound to CSBG.

After OCs are stopped, CSBG-bound cortisol levels may remain elevated and free progesterone levels may be decreased until CSBG levels return to normal. The first cycles after OCs are stopped and even in early pregnancy may be associated with progesterone deficiency. In one study, dehydroepiandrosterone sulfate (DHEAS) levels decreased 30 percent in women using OCs containing 0.15 mg desogestrel. In another study, DHEAS levels decreased 30 to 40 percent in women using OCs containing 0.4 to 1 mg norethindrone but not in women using OCs containing 0.15 mg LNG.

Causal Factors

OCs cause an increase in CSBG (transcortin) because of the estrogen component. High doses of estrogens alter the hepatic metabolism of corticosteroids.

Management

No treatment is required for mild elevations in serum cortisol during OC use, though the slight elevation of free cortisol may result in relief of arthritis and other inflammatory conditions.

Steroid-sensitive patients may experience a worsening of their conditions when they discontinue OCs. Menstrual cycles and early pregnancy may be characterized by progesterone deficiency, despite apparently normal progesterone levels.

References: 214, 216

THYROID CHANGES

Clinical Information

OC use causes increased serum levels of bound thyroxin (T_4), but unbound T_4 and thyroid stimulating hormone (TSH) are unchanged. The increase is due to estrogen, which causes an increase in thyroid binding globulin (TBG). A mild clinical hypothyroid state may be hidden by apparently normal T_4 levels while OCs are being used and for several months after they are discontinued. Untreated hypothyroidism is associated with anovulation and, if pregnancy occurs, a high rate of spontaneous abortion (Ref 246). No association between thyroid disease and OC use per se was found by either the RCGP study (Ref 120) or the Walnut Creek study (Ref 334).

Thyroid nodules and thyroid neoplasia are not related to OC use but may be detected for the first time in women taking OCs because of the high incidence in this age group. The incidence of malignancy in thyroid nodules is high; 20 percent of active (hot) nodules and 70 percent of inactive (cold) nodules are malignant in women of reproductive age. Thyroid neoplasms are slow-growing and rarely metastasize.

Causal Factors

During OC use, increased amounts of TBG are produced due to the effect of estrogen. As a result, thyroid blood studies are altered, including:

- Decreased free T_3 resin uptake
- Increased circulating total thyroid hormone as measured by:
  - Protein-bound iodine (PBI)
  - T_4 by column
  - T_4 by radioimmunoassay

There may be no change in free T_4 concentration.

Management

OC users who exhibit clinical hypothyroid symptoms and users of OCs during the six months previous to exhibiting such symptoms should be evaluated and treated, though serum tests may not be accurate. TSH levels may help establish a diagnosis.

The thyroid gland should be palpated and deep tendon reflexes should be checked before OCs are started; examinations should be repeated annually thereafter. All patients with thyroid nodules should receive further evaluation, including radioactive iodine scans.

References: 120, 246, 334

NOTES

#14 Gastrointestinal System

Nausea/Vomiting
Abdominal Bloating
Abdominal Pain
Gastrointestinal Ulcers
Oral Lesions

NAUSEA/VOMITING

Clinical Information

Nausea and vomiting are most severe during the first cycles of OC use and usually disappear with time. Symptoms occur more often in women who have experienced marked nausea during pregnancy. Nausea that occurs several hours after meals may be due to hypoglycemia. Vomiting and diarrhea were reported by 34 percent of women with "pill failure" who had not missed taking their OCs.

Causal Factors

Nausea similar to morning sickness of early pregnancy is common in OC users and is related to the estrogen dose. Hypoglycemia is related to the progestin component of OCs. Most nausea is caused by gastrointestinal disease and not by OC use.

Management

Patients may relieve nausea by taking their OCs with food or at bedtime.

If symptoms persist after the third cycle of OC use or are unusually severe, such patients should be switched to OCs with less estrogenic activities and advised to follow diets low in carbohydrates.

Symptoms of hypoglycemia should be relieved by switching patients to OCs with less progestational activities.

14.

References: 83, 87, 391

ABDOMINAL BLOATING

Clinical Information

Bloating or swelling of the lower abdomen is common in women having regular ovulatory cycles and is part of the premenstrual complex, which also includes:

- Swelling of the extremities
- Headache
- Irritability
- Occasional nausea

Causal Factors

Premenstrual fluid retention in women not taking OCs is due to the rebound sodium and water retention that follows a decrease in progesterone secretion by the corpus luteum. Progesterone enhances sodium and water excretion, possibly by blocking aldosterone action, while estrogen and androgen cause the sodium and water retention. The progestin component of OCs derived from 19-nor-testosterone does not cause sodium and water excretion as progesterone does but may instead cause fluid retention due to the androgenic activity of either the progestin or estrogen component.

Abdominal bloating during the period that active OCs are taken may also be caused by a reduction in bowel peristalsis due to the smooth muscle relaxing effect of progestin.

Management

Patients may be switched to OCs with lower estrogenic activities if other fluid retention symptoms are present or to OCs with lower progestational activities if symptoms of progestin and/or androgen excess are present (Table 5).

References: 81, 83

ABDOMINAL PAIN

Clinical Information
Abdominal pain includes symptoms identified as:
- Abdominal cramping
- Epigastric distress
- Gastritis
- Intestinal flu

Gastritis due to OCs may appear in the first cycle of OC use and with the first OCs in subsequent cycles. This should lessen with continued use.

Acute gastritis unrelated to OC use may occur at any time.

Very severe pain may be the result of thrombosis of the mesenteric artery or to other diseases unrelated to OC use (see Section #12).

Causal Factors
Women with nutritionally limited diets frequently complain of:
- Epigastric distress
- Stomach pain
- Abdominal cramps

Intestinal flu (gastric influenza) may be one of several viral infections that occurs more frequently in OC users. It is related to estrogen dosage and is reported almost twice as often (1.89 times) in OC users as nonusers. Symptoms of intestinal flu are usually described as:
- An acute attack of diarrhea
- Vomiting
- Fever
- Malaise

Management
OC users may prevent gastritis by taking their pills with food and by using common antacid preparations.

If symptoms persist or first appear after the OC has been used for some time, physicians should consider other causes of abdominal pain, such as:

- Torsion of intestines, ovaries, or a fibroid
- Cholecystitis
- Myocardial infarction (MI)
- Thrombosis of an abdominal vein or artery
- Reflux of gastric contents due to hiatal hernia
- Appendicitis
- Pancreatitis
- Renal calculi
- Pelvic inflammatory disease (PID)

After these conditions have been eliminated as possibilities, a switch to an OC with a lower dose of estrogen and progestin may relieve gastritis.

GASTROINTESTINAL ULCERS

Duodenal and Gastric Ulcers

Duodenal ulcers are six to 12 times less common in women than in men. The incidence of duodenal ulcers is further reduced by pregnancy and is decreased by 40 percent in OC users. The reduced incidence is related to the progestin dose.

The difference in incidence of gastric ulcers is insignificant between OC users and nonusers.

Reference: 356

Ulcerative Colitis and Regional Enteritis

Ulcerative colitis and regional enteritis (Crohn's disease) may change in severity during pregnancy. However, no direct relationship to steroids is known.

The incidence of ulcerative colitis was increased twofold and regional enteritis by 40 percent in OC users in one study. In a study of hospitalized patients, the risk of regional enteritis was increased eight times in women who used OCs for five years or longer.

In another study of patients attending clinics for bowel disease, a significant excess of women with

Crohn's disease confined to the colon had taken OCs during the year before developing symptoms (63 percent) compared to women with small intestinal Crohn's disease (24 percent) and ulcerative colitis (nine percent).

A prospective study from the Oxford Family Planning Association also found an increase in ulcerative colitis and regional enteritis in OC users. The risk of Crohn's disease appears to increase with years of OC use, though the incidence returned to normal four years after discontinuing OCs.

Smoking also was shown to increase the risks of both regional enteritis and ulcerative colitis.

Several authors have noted that blood-stained diarrhea occurring in association with OC use may be due to vascular damage to the colon, resulting in ischemic colitis. Complete recovery was usual for these patients after they discontinued OC use. Patients who experience bloody diarrhea for the first time while taking OCs should discontinue use.

Patients with ulcerative colitis and regional enteritis should be observed closely and OCs stopped if increasing severity of disease or frequency of attacks occurs.

References: 104, 141, 230, 339, 356, 463

ORAL LESIONS

Several surveys and case reports indicate an increased incidence of gingivitis in OC users. One large survey found an increase of about 30 percent in periapical abscess, chronic gingivitis, and mouth ulcers, conditions unrelated to OC dose. This rate increase may have been the result of over-reporting.

Hyperplasia of the gums (gingivitis) also occurs more frequently in pregnant women, but the cause is unknown. Mouth ulcers due to the herpes simplex virus are more common in OC users, as are several types of viral infections.

Salivary calculi are increased 76 percent in OC users, but the total incidence is small (less than 0.3 per 1,000 women per years of use).

If these conditions recur, patients may be switched to OCs with reduced doses of estrogen and progestin or they may discontinue OC use.

References: 356

#15 Integumentary System

Hair Changes
Acne Vulgaris
Chloasma
Melanoma
Rash and Itching
Lupus Erythematosus
Telangiectasias

HAIR CHANGES

Clinical Information

Excessive facial and body hair are commonly diminished in OC users because androgens of ovarian origin and serum free testosterone are suppressed during OC use.

Changes in facial and body hair due to these variations in hormone levels include loss of scalp hair and male pattern hair growth on the face and body.

Hair loss (alopecia) is usually not related to OC use. Hypothyroidism usually leads to thinning and brittleness rather than loss of hair. Alopecia areata (i.e., patchy baldness) is a symptom of secondary syphilis. Loss of hair may also result from:

- Nervous disorders
- Cancer chemotherapy
- Severe illness

Hypothyroidism may cause:

- Thinning of scalp hair
- Hair loss on scalp and body
- Dry skin

15. Loss of scalp hair (male pattern baldness) occurring during use of OCs with high androgen levels is usually due to neoplasms and not OCs.

High androgen levels can cause an increase or darkening of facial and body hair, especially on the:
- Chin
- Chest
- Abdomen (below the umbilicus)

ACNE VULGARIS

Clinical Information

Acne is the result of increased sebum production associated with blocked and infected pores. Testosterone, the most active androgen, is produced directly in the ovary and indirectly by peripheral conversion of weaker androgens produced by the adrenal glands.

Increased androgen levels cause increased sebum production, leading to pimples and acne. Abnormal circulating androgen levels are present in 90 percent of young women with acne.

Insulin resistance has recently been recognized as the cause of increased serum androgen levels and anovulation in 30 percent of women formerly thought to have polycystic ovarian syndrome.

Causal Factors

Most OCs are androgenic to some degree (Table 5). Androgenic symptoms may result from:
- A decrease in sex hormone binding globulin (SHBG)
- Failure to suppress endogenous ovarian androgen production
- Occupancy by progestin of androgen binding sites on serum binding globulins
- Inherent androgenic activity of a particular progestin

A decrease in SHBG may occur with some OCs due to low estrogenic activities. This decrease allows increased circulating amounts of free androgen of adrenal or ovarian origin. Low estrogenic activity rather than high inherent androgenic activity is the probable cause of most androgenic symptoms if they begin during OC use.

Management

OCs with progestins that have low androgenic-to-progestin activity ratios (such as desogestrel, ethynodiol diacetate, gestodene, and norethindrone) or OCs with moderate-to-high estrogen contents and activities increase SHBG and are most likely to result in relief from acne. Ortho Tri-Cyclen®, a triphasic norgestimate OC containing 35 mcg ethinyl estradiol (EE), has been specifically approved for treatment of acne (see Section #6, *Treatment of Acne Vulgaris*). If androgenic symptoms worsen instead, there is a possibility that the androgen increase is coming from the adrenal glands or from an adrenal or ovarian neoplasm.

Androgenic symptoms ordinarily disappear when a switch is made to an OC with greater estrogenic activity. The possibility that androgenic symptoms are the result of androgenic activity of the OC may be determined by switching the patient to an OC with less androgenic activity but equal estrogenic activity (Table 5).

Diet changes and diligent cleansing of the skin will frequently result in relief of acne.

The rate of body hair growth should slow and sebum should be markedly decreased within one month following an effective switch in OCs. Actual loss of new body hair growth may take up to one year to occur.

If sebum production and body hair growth fail to decrease, patients should be evaluated for other causes of increased androgen, such as ovarian or adrenal tumor or hyperplasia.

Hyperthyroidism as a cause of scalp and body hair loss requires evaluation by appropriate tests, although thyroid tests may be abnormal during OC use.

References: 75, 83, 141, 309, 333, 337, 402

CHLOASMA

Clinical Information

Chloasma, also called hyperpigmentation or mask of pregnancy, is an entirely benign condition characterized by the appearance on the skin of brown patches of irregular shapes and sizes.

Chloasma occurs more frequently in women exposed to excessive sunlight and who normally have dark complexions.

Causal Factors

The cause of chloasma is unknown, but it may be related to increased melanocyte stimulating hormone (melatonin) induced by OC use.

Some chloasma appears to be caused by the estrogen component of OCs. In a comparative trial of OCs containing norethindrone and norgestrel, the latter, with more androgenic and equal amounts of estrogens and more progesterone potency, produced a higher incidence of chloasma.

Management

Chloasma must be distinguished from other causes of hyperpigmentation, such as adrenal failure (Addison's disease). A switch to an OC with less estrogenic activity often results in a decrease in pigmentation (Table 5), though the pigmentation may never entirely disappear.

References: 83, 87, 141, 333, 364

MELANOMA

Early reports of a possible 1.7 to 1.8 relative risk of melanoma in OC users have been refuted. Three subsequent reports involving 612 female patients found no relationship between OC use and melanoma in the U.S., Australia, or western Canada. These reports also found no relationship between melanoma and estrogen replacement but did find a significantly decreased incidence of melanoma in women who had experienced five or more births and in women who had undergone bilateral oophorectomy.

References: 127, 148, 169, 473

RASH AND ITCHING

Clinical Information

Symptoms of rash and itching may also be described as:

- Skin eruptions
- Urticaria
- Exanthema
- Pruritus

Rashes and itching are common complaints and may be due to many causes other than OCs, including insect bites and contact dermatitis.

Causal Factors

Rash and itching may occur in women who are allergic to the inactive ingredients used in OCs or to dyes used to add color (see Table 4 for a list of inactive ingredients). Lactose is used as a filler in many OCs. Rash or itching due to drug idiosyncrasy occurs in a small percentage of OC users as with any drug and is usually due to the progestin component.

Management

Symptoms of rash and itching may indicate an underlying pathological condition, such as cholestatic jaundice or hepatitis (see Section #16).

If rash and itching are due to OC use, they may be due to either inactive ingredients or the progestin component. Patients may experience relief by switching to OCs with different inactive ingredients or different progestins (Table 5).

Reference: 83

LUPUS ERYTHEMATOSUS

Estrogen may cause cutaneous lupus to progress to systemic lupus by promoting B-cell hyper-responsiveness and inducing or increasing autoimmunity (Ref 140). Testosterone appears to have a protective effect in lupus. Women with longstanding treatment-refractory lupus who are taking OCs may show significant symptomatic improvement and greater treatment responsiveness if they discontinue OC use. At least one clinician advises women with lupus erythematosus (LE) not to take OCs or estrogen (Ref 140).

TELANGIECTASIAS

Clinical Information

Skin changes may include telangiectasias (liver spots) or spider nevi.

Telangiectasias may be hereditary or may be a manifestation of generalized purpura or of a hematological disorder.

Spider nevi are characterized by a central vessel that may be seen when a glass slide is placed over the lesion. These are usually found in the upper part of the body.

Causal Factors

Telangiectasias are due to capillary dilatation and fragility. Spider nevi occur with cirrhosis of the liver. These conditions are thought to be related to the elevated estrogen levels that occur in some OC users. They also occur more frequently with age.

Management

When telangiectasias are of recent origin and are not associated with evidence of bleeding elsewhere (such as in joints and extremities), they may be due to excess estrogenic activity. In such cases, patients should be switched to OCs with lower estrogenic activities (Table 5).

References: 81, 83

#16 Hepatic/Biliary Systems

Cholecystitis/Cholelithiasis
Cholestatic Jaundice and Pruritus
Hepatoma and Malignant Liver Tumor
Hepatic Infarction and Thrombosis

CHOLECYSTITIS/CHOLELITHIASIS

Gallbladder Disease

Earlier studies have reported an increased lifetime relative risk of gallbladder surgery in users of oral contraceptives and estrogens. More recent studies, however, have shown that the relative risk of developing gallbladder disease among oral contraceptive users may be minimal. The recent findings of minimal risk may be related to the use of oral contraceptive formulations containing lower hormonal doses of estrogens and progestogens.

-FDA Package Insert Labeling

Clinical Information

Changes in the gallbladder may include cholecystitis (inflammation) or cholelithiasis (gallstones).

The incidence of surgically confirmed cholecystitis and cholelithiasis is twice as high in OC users as in nonusers in the U.S.; the same relationship was not found in England. A retrospective study in the U.S. found an annual attack rate of 158 per 100,000 OC users; a British prospective study found a rate of 68 per 100,000 OC users, not significantly different from the rate found for nonusers.

Two studies from Australia and the U.S. found that the risk of developing gallstones was highest in young women and was low or nonexistent in older women. The U.S. study found the relative risk (RR) of all women developing gallstones was:

Age/Years	Relative Risk	Confidence Interval
15 to 19	3.10	2.7 to 3.6
20 to 24	1.50	1.4 to 1.6
25 to 44	1.15	1.1 to 1.2

16.

The actual incidence in OC users was:

Age/Years	Incidence Per 1,000 Women/Years
15 to 29	16.2
20 to 24	26.2
25 to 29	31.8
30 to 34	36.3
35 to 39	45.3
40 to 44	52.4

In one study, an increased risk appeared after two years of OC use and doubled after four or five years of use. In another study, an increased risk was apparent between six and 12 months of use. Obstructive jaundice due to cholelithiasis occurs only rarely and is accompanied by other symptoms.

There are no data to suggest that prior gallbladder disease is a contraindication to OC use.

Causal Factors

Reduced cholesterol excretion, possibly caused by progestins, results in cholesterol precipitation in the gallbladder so that gallstones are formed. Some studies have found an increased risk of surgically confirmed gallbladder disease in users of estrogens. Sonographic studies have found no effect of OCs on gallbladder function.

Management

The onset of cholecystitis and cholelithiasis is characterized by acute abdominal pain. Patients with abdominal pain require complete medical evaluation. Other conditions with similar symptoms may be fatal.

The risk of cholecystitis and cholelithiasis and the incidence of repeated attacks of these diseases may be reduced by use of OCs with low estrogen and progestin doses.

References: 21, 35, 36, 39, 109, 110, 141, 330, 331, 356, 373, 405

CHOLESTATIC JAUNDICE AND PRURITUS

Liver Function
 If jaundice develops in any woman receiving oral contraceptives, the medication should be discontinued. Steroid hormones may be poorly metabolized in patients with impaired liver function.

-FDA Package Insert Labeling

Clinical Information
 Causes of cholestatic jaundice include:
- Hepatocanalicular jaundice
- Cholangiolitic hepatitis
- Obstructive jaundice

 Cholestatic jaundice in OC users is rare, though some individuals and ethnic groups (e.g., Scandinavians and Chileans) appear to be more susceptible. Approximately 50 percent of OC jaundice occurs during the first cycle of OC use and 90 percent during the first six cycles.
 When jaundice of pregnancy occurs, it is more likely to recur in subsequent pregnancies.
 Symptoms of jaundice and pruritus are the cardinal signs of cholestatic jaundice.
 Laboratory findings include:
- An increase in alkaline phosphatase
- Normal transaminase (15 percent show moderate elevation)
- Cholestasis seen in liver biopsy, with little or no parenchymal injury or partial inflammation

 After OCs are discontinued, tests of liver function and hepatic histology become normal and jaundice usually disappears completely within two to three months.

Causal Factors
 Cholestatic jaundice may be the sequel of infectious hepatitis or it may follow use of:
- Methyltestosterone or other androgens
- Sulfonamides
- Thiouracil
- Triacetyloleandomycin (TAO)

Both the estrogen and progestin components of OCs can cause liver dysfunction. Synthesis and/or release of gamma-glutamyl transpeptidase (GGTP) appear to be decreased during OC use and during the second half of pregnancy. The use of OCs with TAO and perhaps other drugs associated with cholestatic jaundice is additive and possibly synergistic. Severe alcoholic cirrhosis but not primary biliary cirrhosis affects the metabolism of medroxyprogesterone acetate (MPA). The effect on the metabolism of other contraceptive steroids is uncertain.

Management

If jaundice occurs, OCs should be stopped until its cause can be determined. If an etiology other than OC use can be determined, OCs may be restarted after liver function tests return to normal or three months after clinical symptoms disappear. If symptoms recur, OCs should be permanently discontinued.

Because these conditions may worsen during pregnancy, it is important that symptomatic patients who have discontinued OC use avoid pregnancy by using other contraceptive methods. Medical treatment of cholestasis may consist of parenteral vitamin K, cholestyramine to bind bile acids and estrogens in the gastrointestinal lumen, and phenobarbital to reduce pruritus.

References: 83, 109, 110, 141, 158, 330, 331, 335, 356

HEPATOMA AND MALIGNANT LIVER TUMOR

Hepatic Neoplasia

Benign hepatic adenomas are associated with oral contraceptive use, although the incidence of benign tumors is rare in the United States. Indirect calculations have estimated the attributable risk to be in the range of 3.3 cases per 100,000 for users, a risk that increases after four or more years of use. Rupture of rare, benign, hepatic adenomas may cause death through intra-abdominal hemorrhage. Studies in the United States and Britain have shown an increased risk of developing hepatocellular carcinoma in long-term (greater than eight years) oral contraceptive users. However, these cancers are extremely rare in the United States and the attributable risk (the excess incidence) of liver cancer in oral contraceptive users is less than one per one million users.

-FDA Package Insert Labeling

Clinical Information

Liver changes associated with OC use may include:

- Hepatoma (benign adenoma)
- Cholangiocarcinoma
- Hepatocellular carcinoma

A 1995 meta-analysis estimated the risk of liver cancer in nonusers of OCs from ages 20 to 54 to be 20 per 100,000 women. For women who used OCs for eight years, an estimated additional 41 liver cancers developed (Ref 368). However, population-based data do not support evidence of a measurable effect of OCs on primary liver cancer. Hepatic cancer rates rose in Japan, during a time when OCs were not used (Ref 470).

Benign hepatic adenomas have been found to be associated with OC use. One study showed that high-potency OCs were associated with a higher risk of hepatocellular adenoma, particularly in women older than age 30. Although they are benign, hepatic adenomas may rupture and cause death through intra-abdominal hemorrhage. This has been reported in short- as well as long-term OC users. Two studies relate risk to duration of use, the risk being much greater after four or more years of OC use. While hepatic adenoma is a rare lesion, it should be considered in women with symptoms of:

- Abdominal pain or tenderness
- Abdominal mass
- Shock

Benign adenomas and malignant liver tumors are rare events, with a combined incidence of between one and four per one million women. Women who use OCs for five years appear to have a five times greater chance of developing hepatomas. Two 1986 studies found that the RR of hepatocellular carcinoma was 4.4 (7.2 if patients with histories of hepatitis B were excluded) to 20.1 after eight years of OC use. There was little or no increased risk for short-term use; nor was there an increase in cholangiocarcinoma.

Clinically significant benign liver tumors are usually palpable; malignant tumors are always palpable. Symptoms may mimic those of:

- Cholecystitis
- Peptic ulcer
- Ischemic heart disease

A liver bruit may be present. Acute abdominal pain and signs of intraperitoneal blood indicate that rupture of the tumor has occurred. Rupture is the principal cause of death in cases of benign tumors.

Hepatocellular carcinoma is a rare disease (115 cases in OC users and nonusers ages 15 to 49 in 1979 in the U.S.). In underdeveloped countries, the occurrence may be 10 to 20 times higher. A few cases of hepatocellular carcinoma have been reported among OC users, but the relationship of OCs to this malignancy is not known.

When compared to nonusers, OC users with malignant liver tumors:

- Are younger
- Have normal α-fetoprotein (AFP) levels
- Have more vascular tumors

Survival times are longer for OC users, with a 50-percent survival of 4.8 years compared to 1.8 years for nonusers. This is similar to the relationship between breast cancer and OCs, in which OC users had a longer survival time than nonusers.

Causal Factors

It has been proposed that estrogens are important in the genesis of liver tumors by impairing biliary secretions and causing decreased blood flow. However, testosterone and androgenic drugs are reported to increase the incidence of hepatoma in both men and women. Infection from the hepatitis B virus is strongly associated with hepatocellular carcinoma.

Management

Acute abdominal pain and signs of intraperitoneal blood constitute an emergency requiring hospitalization and surgical exploration. All patients taking OCs should have the edge of the liver palpated at their annual or semi-annual examinations. This becomes more important after OCs have been taken for several years. If a liver mass is discovered, OCs must be stopped immediately.

If a mass is palpable, selective hepatic angiography may demonstrate a tumor, though radiological methods cannot distinguish a malignant tumor from a benign one. Marked increases in serum alkaline phosphatase are characteristic of malignant tumors; transaminase and α-fetoprotein levels are usually normal.

Benign liver tumors regress in size after OCs are stopped, so that surgery may not be necessary. Because benign tumors may grow rapidly during pregnancy, it is essential that patients with benign liver tumors who discontinue OCs use alternative contraceptive methods. The size of a tumor may be followed by ultrasonography.

Women with histories of the hepatitis B virus should perhaps not use steroidal contraception, due to the increased risk of hepatocellular carcinoma.

References: 21, 98, 109, 110, 183, 262, 286, 288, 289, 330, 343, 368, 470

HEPATIC INFARCTION AND THROMBOSIS

Clinical Information

Only one U.S. case of hepatic common artery thrombosis with subsequent hepatic infarction has been reported. Other reported hepatic vascular complications in OC users include:

- Budd-Chiari syndrome (hepatic vein thrombosis)
- Portal vein thrombosis

- Periportal sinusoidal dilatation
- Hepatic arteriole (intimal hyperplasia)
- Focal hemorrhagic necrosis

Management

The liver should be palpated at each examination.

References: 6, 188, 189, 508, 509

17.

TABLE 1 – Beneficial Effects of Oral Contraceptives

Condition or Disease	Percent Reductions Compared to Nonusers	References
Pregnancy		
Term vaginal delivery	99%	306
Term cesarean section	99%	306
Spontaneous abortion, D & C	99%	306
Ectopic pregnancy	99%	306
Menstrual Disorders		
Dysmenorrhea	63%	356
Menopausal symptoms	72%	356
Menorrhagia	48%	356
Irregular menstruation	35%	356
Intermenstrual bleeding	28%	356
Premenstrual tension	29%	356
Reproductive Organ Neoplasm		
Fibrocystic and fibroadenoma breast disease	50 to 75%	43, 303, 305, 308, 358
Breast biopsies	50%	304

Benign ovarian cysts	65%	358, 461, 505
Uterine fibroma*	59%	356
Ovarian cancer	40%	56, 478
Endometrial cancer	50%	42, 61, 205, 209, 381, 382, 477
Other Reproductive Disorders		
Endometriosis*	50%	42, 109, 356
Pelvic inflammatory disease- all cases*	10 to 70%	374
Pelvic inflammatory disease- hospitalized cases*	10 to 70%	110, 374
Toxic shock syndrome	60%	146, 190
Uterine retroversion	24%	356
Other Symptoms		
Rheumatoid arthritis	50%	242, 356, 482
Iron deficiency anemia	45%	356, 461, 473
Duodenal ulcer	40%	356
Sebaceous cysts	24%	356
Acne	16%	356

*These conditions may have a significant adverse effect on future reproductive capabilities.

TABLE 2 – Effectiveness and Mortality of Contraceptive Methods

Method	Pregnancies Per 100 Women/Years All Ages [1]		Estimated Annual Deaths Due to Contraceptive Method and/or Pregnancy [2] Per 100,000 Women/Years by Age [2]					
	Lowest Expected	Typical	15-19	20-24	25-29	30-34	35-39	40-44
No Contraception	85	85	6	5	7	14	19	22
Surgical Sterilization [3] (Tubal ligation)	0.2	0.4	4	4	4	4	4	4
Combination Oral Contraceptives								
Non-smokers	0.1	3	1	1	1	2	4	3
Smokers	0.1	3	2	2	2	11	13	59
Progestin-Only Oral Contraceptives	0.5	3	1	1	1	1	1	1
Progestin Injections								
Medroxyprogesterone acetate (MPA)	0.3	0.3	1	1	1	1	1	1
Norethindrone enanthanate (NET)	0.4	0.4	1	1	1	1	1	1
Progestin Implants								
Levonorgestrel (LNG)	0.3	0.3	1	1	1	1	1	1

Intrauterine Devices

Progestasert ®	2.0	1	1	1	1	1	2	1
ParaGard® T 380A	0.8	1	1	1	1	1	1	1

Barrier Methods

Diaphragm Cap	6	18	1 - 2	1 - 2	1 - 2	1 - 4	1 - 6	1 - 7
Condoms	2	12	1 - 3	1 - 3	1 - 4	1 - 7	1 - 11	1 - 12
Aerosol foam, jelly, cream, tablets	3	21	1 - 3	1 - 3	1 - 4	1 - 7	1 - 11	1 - 12
Sponge								
Parous women	9	28	1 - 2	1 - 2	1 - 3	1 - 6	1 - 8	1 - 10
Nulliparous women	6	18	1 - 2	1 - 2	1 - 2	1 - 4	1 - 6	1 - 7

Periodic Abstinence (rhythm)

Periodic Abstinence (rhythm)	1-9	20	1 - 2	1 - 2	1 - 2	1 - 4	1 - 16	1 - 16

1. Reference: 433, 434
2. Reference: 430
3. Reference: 315

In a comparative study of 1,437 women using the sponge vs. diaphragm and a study of 1,394 women using the cervical cap vs. diaphragm the 12 months failure rate was diaphragm 5.2 and 6.9%, cervical cap 11.4%, sponge 11.7%. Failure rates increased to 26.4% for the cap and 20% for the sponge among parous users. The failure rate for condoms was estimated at 2.7%. J. Trussel, Office of Population Research, Princeton University, 1993.

TABLE 3 – Biological Activity of Oral Contraceptive Components

Class Compound	Progestational Activity[1]	Estrogenic Activity[2]	Androgenic Activity[3]	Endometrial Activity[4]	Andro:Prog Activity Ratio[5]
Progestins[6]					
19 Nor-Testosterone Progestins					
Estrane					
Norethindrone	1.0	1.0	1.0	1.0	1.0
Norethindrone acetate	1.2	1.5	1.6	0.4	1.3
Ethynodiol diacetate	1.4	3.4	0.6	0.4	0.4
5(10) Estrane					
Norethynodrel	0.3	8.3	0	0	0
Gonane					
Levonorgestrel	5.3	0	8.3	5.1	1.6
dl-Norgestrel	2.6	0	4.2	2.6	1.6
Norgestimate	1.3	0	1.9	1.2	1.5
Desogestrel	9.0	0	3.4	8.7	0.4
Gestodene	12.6	0	8.6	12.6	0.7

Pregnane Progestins

Chlormadinone acetate	1.0	0	0	NA	0
Megestrol acetate	0.4	0	0	NA	0
Medroxyprogesterone acetate	0.3	0	0	NA	0

Estrogens[7]

Ethinyl estradiol	0	100	0	0	0
Mestranol	0	67	0	0	0

1. Based on amount required to induce vacuoles in human endometrium. Reference: 68. Desogestrel, gestodene, levonorgestrel and norgestimate based on oral stimulation of endometrium in immature estrogen-primed rabbits relative to levonorgestrel = 5.3. Reference: 321.

2. Comparative potency based on oral rat vaginal epithelium assay. (Norethindrone = 0.2 when ethinyl estradiol = 100. Reference: 197).

3. Comparative potency (oral) based on rat ventral prostate assay. (Norethindrone = 1.0 when methyltestosterone = 50. Reference: 422). (Levonorgestrel and desogestrel relative to norethindrone = 1.0. Reference:214) (Norgestimate, relative to levonorgestrel = 8.3. Reference: 321) and (Gestodene relative to levonorgestrel = 8.3 Reference 101).

4. Based on estimation of amount required to suppress bleeding for 20 days in 50% of women. Reference: 416.

5. Based on oral and animal assays. Actual activity in women may be different and will be modified by the dose of estrogen.

6. Calculated on the basis of norethindrone = 1.0 in activity.

7. Calculated on the basis of ethinyl estradiol = 100 in activity.

143

TABLE 4 – Composition and Identification of Oral Contraceptives

Name	Progestin	mg	Estrogen	mcg	Manufacturer	Color A/IA[5]	Inactive Ingredient[8]
Monophasic							
Alesse	Levonorgestrel	0.1	E. estradiol[3]	20	Wyeth	P (G)	d
Brevicon	Norethindrone	0.5	E. estradiol	35	Searle	Bl (O)	a
Demulen	Ethy. diacetate[1]	1.0	E. estradiol	50	Searle	W (P)	b
Demulen 1/35	Ethy. diacetate	1.0	E. estradiol	35	Searle	W (Bl)	b
Desogen	Desogestrel	0.15	E. estradiol	30	Organon	W (G)	c
Genora 1/35	Norethindrone	1.0	E. estradiol	35	Rugby	Bl (Pe)	a
Genora 1/50	Norethindrone	1.0	Mestranol	50	Rugby	W (Pe)	a
Levlen	Levonorgestrel	0.15	E. estradiol	30	Berlex	Pe (P)	d
Levora	Levonorgestrel	0.15	E. estradiol	30	Watson	W (Pe)	a
Loestrin 1.5/30	Nor. acetate[2]	1.5	E. estradiol	30	Parke-Davis	G (Br)[6]	e
Loestrin 1/20	Nor. acetate	1.0	E. estradiol	20	Parke-Davis	W(Br)[6]	c
Lo/Ovral	Norgestrel	0.3	E. estradiol	30	Wyeth	W (P)	d
Mircette	Desogestrel	0.15	E. estradiol	20	Organon	W(G)Y[7]	c
Modicon	Norethindrone	0.5	E. estradiol	35	Ortho	W (G)	f
Necon 0.5/35	Norethindrone	0.5	E. estradiol	35	Watson	LY (W)	a
Necon 1/35	Norethindrone	1.0	E. estradiol	35	Watson	Y (W)	a
Necon 1/50M	Norethindrone	1.0	Mestranol	50	Watson	Bl (W)	a
Nelova 1/50M	Norethindrone	1.0	Mestranol	50	Warner Chilcott	LBl(W)	a
Nelova 1/35E	Norethindrone	1.0	E. estradiol	35	Warner Chilcott	DY(W)	a

Name	Progestin	Dose	Estrogen	Dose	Manufacturer	Color	
Nelova 0.5/35E	Norethindrone	0.5	E. estradiol	35	Warner Chilcott	Y (W)	a
Nordette	Levonorgestrel	0.15	E. estradiol	30	Wyeth	Pe (P)	d
Norethin 1/35	Norethindrone	1.0	E. estradiol	35	Roberts	W (B)	b
Norethin 1/50M	Norethindrone	1.0	Mestranol	50	Roberts	W (B)	b
Norinyl 1/35	Norethindrone	1.0	E. estradiol	35	Searle	G (O)	a
Norinyl 1/50	Norethindrone	1.0	Mestranol	50	Searle	W (O)	a
Norlestrin 1/50	Nor. acetate	1.0	E. estradiol	50	Parke-Davis	Y (W)(Br)6	e
Ortho-Cept	Desogestrel	0.15	E. estradiol	30	Ortho	O (G)	c
Ortho-Cyclen	Norgestimate	0.25	E. estradiol	35	Ortho	Bl (G)	f
Ortho-Novum 1/35	Norethindrone	1.0	E. estradiol	35	Ortho	O (G)	f
Ortho-Novum 1/50	Norethindrone	1.0	Mestranol	50	Ortho	Y (G)	f
Ovcon 35	Norethindrone	0.4	E. estradiol	35	Mead Johnson	Pe (G)	a
Ovcon 50	Norethindrone	1.0	E. estradiol	50	Mead Johnson	Y (G)	g
Ovral	Norgestrel	0.5	E. estradiol	50	Wyeth	W (P)	d
Zovia 1/35	Ethy. diacetate	1.0	E. estradiol	35	Watson	LP (W)	a
Zovia 1/50	Ethy. diacetate	1.0	E. estradiol	50	Watson	P (W)	a
Multiphasic[4]							
Estrostep	Nor. acetate	1.0(5)	E. estradiol	20(5)	Parke-Davis	W T	e
	Nor. acetate	1.0(7)	E. estradiol	30(7)	Parke-Davis	W S	e
	Nor. acetate	1.0(9)	E. estradiol	35(9)	Parke-Davis	W R (Br)6	e
Jenest	Norethindrone	0.5(7)	E. estradiol	35(7)	Organon	W	f
	Norethindrone	1.0(14)	E. estradiol	35(14)	Organon	Pe (G)	f
Necon 10/11	Norethindrone	0.5(10)	E. estradiol	35(10)	Watson	LY	a
	Norethindrone	1.0(11)	Estradiol	35(11)	Watson	DY	a
Nelova 10/11	Norethindrone	0.5(10)	E. estradiol	35(10)	Warner Chilcott	Y	a
	Norethindrone	1.0(11)	E. estradiol	35(11)	Warner Chilcott	DY (W)	a

→ Continued

TABLE 4 – Composition and Identification of Oral Contraceptives

(continued from previous page)

Name	Progestin	mg	Estrogen	mcg	Manufacturer	Color A/IA[5]	Inactive Ingredient[8]
Ortho-Novum 7/7/7	Norethindrone	0.5(7)	E. estradiol	35(7)	Ortho	W	f
	Norethindrone	0.75(7)	E. estradiol	35(7)	Ortho	LPe	f
	Norethindrone	1.0(7)	E. estradiol	35(7)	Ortho	Pe (G)	f
Ortho-Novum 10/11	Norethindrone	0.5(10)	E. estradiol	35(10)	Ortho	W	f
	Norethindrone	1.0(11)	E. estradiol	35(11)	Ortho	Pe (G)	f
Ortho Tri-Cyclen	Norgestimate	0.180(7)	E. estradiol	35(7)	Ortho	W	f
	Norgestimate	0.215(7)	E. estradiol	35(7)	Ortho	LBl	f
	Norgestimate	0.250(7)	E. estradiol	35(7)	Ortho	Bl (G)	f
Tri-Levlen	Levonorgestrel	0.05(6)	E. estradiol	30(6)	Berlex	Br	d
	Levonorgestrel	0.75(5)	E. estradiol	40(5)	Berlex	W	d
	Levonorgestrel	0.125(10)	E. estradiol	30(10)	Berlex	Y(G)	d
Tri-Norinyl	Norethindrone	0.5(7)	E. estradiol	35(7)	Searle	Bl	a
	Norethindrone	1.0 (9)	E. estradiol	35(9)	Searle	G	a
	Norethindrone	0.5(5)	E. estradiol	35(5)	Searle	Bl (O)	a
Triphasil	Levonorgestrel	0.05(6)	E. estradiol	30(6)	Wyeth	Br	d
	Levonorgestrel	0.075(5)	E. estradiol	40(5)	Wyeth	W	d
	Levonorgestrel	0.125(10)	E. estradiol	30(10)	Wyeth	Y (G)	d
Trivora	Levonorgestrel	0.5(6)	E. estradiol	30(6)	Watson	Bl	a
	Levonorgestrel	0.075(5)	E. estradiol	40(5)	Watson	W	a
	Levonorgestrel	0.125(10)	E. estradiol	30(10)	Watson	P(Pe)	a

Progestin Only

Micronor	Norethindrone	0.35	None	Ortho	G	f
Nor-QD	Norethindrone	0.35	None	Searle	Y	a
Ovrette	Norgestrel	0.075	None	Wyeth	Y	d

1. Ethynodiol diacetate
2. Norethindrone acetate
3. Ethinyl estradiol
4. Multiphasic product: Number in parenthesis = days of each phase
5. Color and shape abbreviations: BI-Blue, Br-Brown, DY-Dark Yellow, G-Green, LPe-Light Peach, LBI-Light Blue, LP-Light Pink, LY-Light Yellow, O-Orange, P-Pink, Pe-Peach or Light Orange, W-White, Y-Yellow, T-Triangular, S-Square, R-Round. Color in parenthesis = inactive tablets.
6. Inactive brown tablets (Br) contain 75 mg ferrous fumarate
7. E. estadiol (Y) 10 mcg for first 5 days of progestin free interval

8. Inactive Ingredient:

   a) Lactose
   Magnesium stearate
   Povidone
   Sodium starch glycolate
     (cornstarch)
     (talc)

   b) Calcium acetate
   Calcium phosphate
   Cornstarch
   Hydrogenated castor oil
   Povidone
     (calcium sulfate)
     (magnesium stearate)
     (sucrose)

   c) Vitamin E
   Cornstarch
   Povidone
   Stearic acid
   Colloidal silicon dioxide
   Lactose
   Hydroxypropyl methylcellulose
   Polyethylene glycol
   Titanium dioxide
   Talc
     (lactose)
     (magnesium stearate)
     (ferric oxide)

   d) Cellulose
   Lactose
   Magnesium stearate
   polacrilin potassium

   e) Acacia
   Lactose
   Magnesium stearate
   Starch
   Confectioner's sugar
   Talc

   f) Lactose
   Magnesium stearate
   Pre-gelatinized starch
   Microcrystalline cellulose

   g) Dibasic calcium phosphate
   Magnesium stearate
   Povidone
   Sodium starch glycolate
     (cornstarch)
     (talc)

TABLE 5 – Contraceptive Pill Activity
[Ranked According to Estrogen Content and Endometrial Potency]

DRUG	ENDOMETRIAL ACTIVITY: % Spotting, and bleeding, in third cycle of use[1]	ESTROGENIC ACTIVITY: mcg Ethinyl Estradiol equivalents per day[2]	PROGESTATIONAL ACTIVITY: mg Norethindrone equivalents per day[3]	ANDROGENIC ACTIVITY: mg Methyltestosterone per 28 days[4]
50 mcg Estrogen				
Ovral	4.5	42	1.3	0.80
Genora/Necon/Nelova/Norethin/ Norinyl/Ortho-Novum 1/50	10.6	32	1.0	0.34
Ovcon 50	11.9	50	1.0	0.34
Norlestrin 1/50	13.6	39	1.2	0.53
Demulen 50/Zovia 1/50	13.9	26	1.4	0.21
Sub-50 mcg Estrogen				
Monophasic				
Lo-Ovral	9.6	25	0.8	0.46
Ovcon 35	11.0	40	0.4	0.15
Desogen/Ortho-Cept	13.1	30	1.5	0.17
Levlen/Levora/Nordette	14.0	25	0.8	0.46
Ortho-Cyclen	14.3	35	0.3	0.18
Genora/Necon/Nelova/Norinyl/ Norethin/Ortho-Novum 1/35	14.7	38	1.0	0.34
Mircette	19.7	22	1.5	0.17
Brevicon/Modicon/Necon/ Nelova 0.5/35	24.6	42	0.5	0.17

Loestrin 1.5/30	25.2	14	1.7	0.80
Alesse	26.5	17	0.5	0.31
Loestrin 1/20	29.7	13	1.2	0.53
Demulen/Zovia 1/35	37.4	19	1.4	0.21
Sub-50 mcg Estrogen				
Multiphasic				
Ortho-Novum 7/7/7	14.5	48	0.8	0.25
Tri-Levlen/Triphasil/Trivora	15.1	28	0.5	0.29
Jenest	17.3	39	0.8	0.28
Necon/Nelova/Ortho-Novum 10/11	17.6	40	0.8	0.25
Ortho Tri-Cyclen	17.7	35	0.3	0.15
Tri-Norinyl	25.5	40	0.7	0.23
Estrostep	26.2	16	1.2	0.53
Progestin-Only				
Ovrette	34.9	0	0.08	0.13
Micronor/Nor-QD	42.3	1	0.12	0.13

1. Information submitted to the United States Food and Drug Administration by the manufacturer. These rates are derived from separate studies conducted by different investigators in several population groups, and therefore, a precise comparison cannot be made, except when randomized comparative studies are used. Randomized comparative studies used are: NDA 18-985 (Ortho 7/7/7 and Jenest vs. Ortho 1 + 35); NDA 19-653 (Ortho-Cyclen vs. Lo-Oval); Syntex laboratories study 17-6288 (Tri-Norinyl and Ortho 10/11 vs. Norinyl 1 + 35).
2. Estrogenic activity of entire tablet - mouse uterine assay. Reference: 59, 86
3. Induction of glycogen vacucles in human endometrium. Reference: 89, 145
4. Rat ventral prostate assay. Reference: 321, 422

TABLE 6 – Effect of Oral Contraceptives and Components on
Serum High Density Lipoprotein Cholesterol (HDL-C) and Low Density Lipoprotein Cholesterol (LDL-C)

PREPARATION / Progestin mg/Estrogen mcg		PERCENT CHANGE FROM CONTROLS							
		STUDY 1*	STUDY 2**	STUDY 3	STUDY 4**	STUDY 5		STUDY 6	
		HDL-C	HDL-C	HDL-C	HDL-C	HDL-C	LDL-C	HDL-C	LDL-C
Estrogen-Only									
Ethinyl estradiol 20		+28	+21	—	—	—	—	—	—
Ethinyl estradiol 50		+25	+46	—	—	—	—	—	—
Progestin-Only									
Levonorgestrel 0.03		—	-2	—	—	—	—	—	—
Medroxyprogesterone acetate 50 IM		-25	-15	—	—	—	—	—	—
Norethindrone 0.35		—	-4	—	—	—	—	—	—
Norethindrone acetate 1		—	-7	—	—	—	—	—	—
Norethindrone acetate 2		—	-11	—	—	—	—	—	—
Combination OC with Norethynodrel									
Enovid E 2.5/100***		—	+26	—	—	—	—	—	—
Combination OC with Norethindrone									
Ortho-Novum/Norinyl 2/100***		+2	-5	—	—	—	—	—	—
Norinyl 1/80***		+5	-6	—	—	—	—	—	—
Ortho-Novum 1/80***		+5	-6	—	—	—	—	—	—
Ortho-Novum/Norinyl 1/50		0	-8	+1.8	—	—	—	—	—
Ortho-Novum/Norinyl 1/35*		—	-11	—	+7.3	-4.1	-5.8	—	—
Brevicon/Modicon 0.5/35		—	-2	—	—	+9.8	-12.1	—	—
Biphasic OC with Norethindrone									
Ortho-Novum 10/11 0.5-1.0/35		—	—	—	—	+4.6	-6.7	—	—

	Study 1	Study 2	Study 3	Study 4	Study 5	Study 6		
Combination OC with Norethindrone Acetate Norlestrin 1 1/20	+1	-10	+1.8	-3.6	—	—	—	—
Combination OC with Ethynodiol Diacetate Demulen 1/30	+10	-13	—	+5.5	—	—	—	—
Combination OC with Levonorgestrel or dl-Norgestrel Ovral 0.5/30	-16	-12	—	-18.2	-15.6	+0.4	—	—
Levlen/Levora/Nordette 0.15/30	—	—	—	—	-4.6	+1.2	—	—
Triphasic OC with Levonorgestrel Tri-Levlen/Triphasil/Trivora 0.15-0.25/30	—	—	—	—	+1.2	-3.3	—	—
Combination OC with Desogestrel Desogen/Ortho-Cept 0.15/30	—	—	—	—	+12.1	-13.8	+12.9	-2.1
Mircette 0.15/20****	—	—	—	—	—	—	+15.1	—
Combination OC with Gestodene Not available in the U.S. 0.75/30	—	—	—	—	—	—	+8.1	-2.5
Combination OC with Norgestimate Ortho-Cyclen 0.25/35	—	—	—	—	—	—	+7.4	+3.4
Triphasic OC with Norgestimate Ortho Tri-Cyclen 0.18-0.25/35	—	—	—	—	—	—	+10.5	+2.1

* Length of OC use 21 days
** Length of OC use variable
*** These pills have been discontinued
**** NDA information cycle 6

Study 1 – References: 219
Study 2 – References: 353
Study 3 – References: 500
Study 4 – References: 471
Study 5 – References: 137
Study 6 – References: 394

TABLE 7 – Ratio: Total Cholesterol Divided By High-Density Lipoprotein Cholesterol

Product	Dose Progestin mg	Dose Estrogen mcg	Number Patients	Ratio	Percent Change From Control	Significance p=
Study 1						
Control	–	–	113	3.2	–	–
Demulen	1	50	6	3.9	+22%	NS
Norlestrin	1 to 2.5	50	8	3.1	– 1%	NS
Ortho-Novum, Norinyl	1 to 2	50 to 100	34	3.3	– 3%	NS
Ovral	0.5	50	20	3.8	+19%	0.01
Study 2						
Control	–	–	293	3.1	–	–
Levlen/Nordette***	0.15	30	206	3.2	+3%	NS
Loestrin	1	20	76	3.1	0	NS
Micronor*	0.35	0	72	3.2	+3%	NS
Ortho-Novum**	1	50	39	3.2	+3%	NS

Study 3						
Control	–	–	5	3.2	–	–
Ovcon 35	0.4	35	10	3.4	+3%	NS
Lo/Ovral	0.3	30	11	3.8	+18%	NS
Study 4						
Control	–	–	642	3.3	–	–
Ortho-Novum	1 to 2	50 to 100	146	3.3	0	NS
Enovid	2.5 to 5	75 to 100	12	2.7	–18%	0.05
Norlestrin	1.0 to 2.5	50	41	3.8	+17%	0.01
Ovral	0.5	50	76	4.3	+32%	0.01
Demulen	1	50	17	3.5	+7%	NS

* Also in this group Neogest equal to Ovrette

** Also in this group Norinyl 1/50, Norlestrin 1/50

*** Equal to Lo/Ovral

Study 1 – Reference: 219   Study 3 – Reference: 500
Study 2 – Reference: 353   Study 4 – Reference: 471

TABLE 8 – Choice of an Initial Oral Contraceptive

After the initial cycles, all patients should be switched to Group 2 through 8 OCs if possible ($\leq$ 35 mcg estrogen, low androgen activity).

Characteristics	Type of OC Indicated	Suggested OC for the Initial Cycles [See Table 9 for OC Groups]
Regular light menses. 2 to 4 days flow: Mild or no cramps.	Low or intermediate endometrial activity.	Group 2, 5-8
Regular moderate menses. 4 to 6 days flow: Moderate cramps	Intermediate endometrial activity.	Group 2, 5, 7
Regular heavy menses. 6-plus days flow: Severe cramps.	High endometrial activity.	Group 13
Irregular and infrequent menses, hypermenorrhea when occurs: Associated acne, oily skin, hirsutism.	Probably polycystic ovarian syndrome. High progestational and low androgenic activity desirable.	Group 2, 6, 12
Irregular menses, hypomenorrhea when occurs: No androgen effects.	If galactorrhea present, possible pituitary adenoma. Skull x-ray or prolactin needed. If no galactorrhea, low estrogen and low progestional activity combination OCs or Multiphasic OCs may be used.	Group 1, 5, 8, barrier and spermicide methods
Smokers-Ages 35 and over	Combination OCs contraindicated	Group 1, barrier and spermicide methods
Nonsmokers-Ages 35 and over	Sub 35 mcg estrogen, intermediate/high progestin, combination OC.	Group 2-4

Weight less than 110 lbs.	Lower estrogen and low progestin dose	Group 5, 7, 8
Weight more than 160 lbs.	High estrogen and progestin activity.	Group 9-13
Progesterone hypersensitivity: History of toxemia, strong family history of hypertension, excessive weight gain, tiredness or varicose veins during pregnancy, depression, excessive premenstrual edema.	Low progestin dose and progestational activity. Monitor blood pressure.	Group 1, 5, 8
Estrogen hypersensitivity: Excessive nausea, edema or hypertension in pregnancy; hypertrophy of the cervix or uterus; uterine fibroids; large or fibrocystic breasts; heavy menses; migraine.	Low estrogenic activity.	Group 1, 3
Conditions predisposing to cardiovascular disease, type II hyperlipidemia (hypercholesterolemia), diabetes mellitus, obesity, smoking more than 15 cigarettes per day, hypertension, varicose veins, thrombophlebitis during pregnancy, family history of cardiovascular disease before age 50.	Combination pills not recommended.	Group 1, barrier and spermicide methods
Surgery planned within one to four weeks.	Combination pills should be stopped.	Group 1, barrier and spermicide methods
Nursing	Oral contraceptives should not be used.	None

TABLE 9 – Oral Contraceptives with Similar Endometrial, Progestational and Androgenic Activities[1]

GROUP	ORAL CONTRACEPTIVES	ESTROGEN AND DOSE	ACTIVITY
#1	Micronor Nor-QD Ovrette	No estrogen	Endometrial: Low Progestational: Low Androgenic: Low
#2	Mircette Desogen Ortho-Cept	22 mcg ethinyl estradiol (Average) 30 mcg ethinyl estradiol 30 mcg ethinyl estradiol	Endometrial: Intermediate Progestational: Intermediate/High Androgenic: Low
#3	Loestrin 1/20 Estrostep* Loestrin 1.5/30	20 mcg ethinyl estradiol 30 mcg ethinyl estradiol (Average) 30 mcg ethinyl estradiol	Endometrial: Low Progestational: Intermediate/High Androgenic: Intermediate/High
#4	Levlen Levora Lo-Ovral Nordette	30 mcg ethinyl estradiol	Endometrial: Intermediate Progestational: Intermediate Androgenic: Intermediate
#5	Tri-Levlen* Triphasil* Trivora* Ovcon 35 Ortho-Cyclen Ortho Tri-Cyclen*	32 mcg ethinyl estradiol (Average) 35 mcg ethinyl estradiol	Endometrial: Intermediate Progestational: Low Androgenic: Low
#6	Demulen 1/35 Zovia 1/35	35 mcg ethinyl estradiol	Endometrial: Low Progestational: High Angdrogenic: Low
#7	Jenest* Necon 10/11* Nelova 10/11* Ortho-Novum 7/7/7* Ortho-Novum 10/11*	35 mcg ethinyl estradiol	Endometrial: Intermediate Progestational: Intermediate Androgenic: Low

#8	Alesse Brevicon Modicon Necon 0.5/35 Nelova 0.5/35 Tri-Norinyl*	20 mcg ethinyl estradiol 35 mcg ethinyl estradiol	Endometrial: Low Progestational: Low Androgenic: Low
#9	Genora 1/35 Necon 1/35 Nelova 1/35 Norethin 1/35E Norinyl 1/35 Ortho-Novum 1/35	35 mcg ethinyl estradiol	Endometrial: Intermediate Progestational: Intermediate Androgenic: Intermediate
#10	Necon 1/50M Norethin 1/50M Norinyl 1/50 Nelova 1/50M Ortho-Novum 1/50 Genora 1/50	50 mcg mestranol	Endometrial: Intermediate Progestational: Intermediate Androgenic: Intermediate
#11	Norlestrin 1/50 Ovcon 1/50	50 mcg ethinyl estradiol	Endometrial: Intermediate Progestational: Intermediate Androgenic: Intermediate
#12	Demulen 1/50 Zovia 1/50	50 mcg ethinyl estradiol	Endometrial: Intermediate Progestational: High Androgenic: Low
#13	Ovral	50 mcg ethinyl estradiol	Endometrial: High Progestational: High Androgenic: High

[1] Arranged by estrogen type and dose, see Table 5 for specific activity.
* Multiphasic

TABLE 10 – Laboratory Changes Associated with OC Use

ESTROGEN RELATED			PROGESTIN RELATED
SERUM INCREASED	**SERUM INCREASED**	**SERUM DECREASED**	**SERUM INCREASED**
Aldosterone	Prolactin	Albumin	Fibrinolysis
Amylase	Prothrombin time	Antithrombin III	Hematocrit
Ceruloplasmin	Renin substrate	Glucose absorption	Insulin
Clotting factors II, VII, VIII, IX, X, XI and prothrombin	(angiotensinogen and renin)	Insulin	Insulin resistance
Cortisol	Sex steroid binding globulin	Prothrombin time	Nitrogen
Erythrocyte sedimentation rate	(testosterone)	Ratio total cholesterol/HDL cholesterol	Ratio total cholesterol and/or HDL-cholesterol/LDL-cholesterol
Fibrinogen	Sodium	Triiodothyronine resin uptake (T_3)	
Free fatty acids	T_4 thyroxine		**SERUM DECREASED**
FSH	Thyroxine binding globulin	**SERUM ALTERED**	Alpha amino nitrogen
Growth hormone	Total lipids	ACTH response	Complement reactive protein
HDL-cholesterol	Transferrin	Bromsulphalein test	HDL-cholesterol
LDL-cholesterol	Triglycerides	Glucose tolerance test	Luteinizing hormone
Protein-bound iodine		Lupus erythematosus cell prep	Triglycerides
Platelet count, aggregation and cohesiveness		Metapyrone test	
Plasmin		**URINE INCREASED**	
Plasminogen		Aldosterone	
		URINE DECREASED	
		Gonadotropins	

ETIOLOGY UNKNOWN

SERUM INCREASED	SERUM INCREASED	SERUM DECREASED	URINE INCREASED
Alkaline phosphatase	Iron	Ascorbic acid	Coproporphyrin
Alpha 1 antitrypsin	Iron binding capacity	Calcium	Delta-aminolevulinic acid
Alpha 1, alpha 2 globulin	Lactate	Cholinesterase	Formiminoglutamic acid
Angiotensin I and II	Leukocyte	Erythrocyte count	excretion after histidine
Antinuclear antibodies	Lipoproteins alpha, beta,	Folate	Porphyrins
Bilirubin	pre-beta, total	Haptoglobin	Xanthurenic acid
Cephalin flocculation	Nucleotidase	Magnesium	
Copper	(5-nucleotidase)	Renin	
Cryofibrinogen	PPT	Vitamin B_{12}	**URINE DECREASED**
Erythrocyte sedimentation rate	Phospholipids	Zinc	
Euglobulin lysis	Plasma volume		17-hydroxy steroids
Formiminoglutamic acid	Pyruvate		17-keto steroids
excretion after histidine	SGOT		Calcium
Gamma glutamyl/	SGPT		Estrogen (-diol, -triol)
transpeptidase	Sodium		Etiocholanolone
Immunoglobulin A	Transaminase		Pregnanediol, (-triol)
Immunoglobulin G	Vitamin A		Tetrahydrocannabinol
Immunoglobulin M			Urobilinogen

TABLE 11 – Relation of Side Effects to Hormone Content

I. REPRODUCTIVE SYSTEM		II. PREMENSTRUAL SYNDROME
ESTROGEN EXCESS Breast cystic changes Cervical extrophy Dysmenorrhea Hypermenorrhea, menorrhagia, and clotting Increase in breast size Mucorrhea Uterine enlargement Uterine fibroid growth ***ESTROGEN DEFICIENCY*** Absence of withdrawal bleeding Bleeding and spotting during pill days 1 to 9 Continuous bleeding and spotting Flow decrease, hypomenorrhea Pelvic relaxation symptoms Vaginitis atrophic	***PROGESTIN EXCESS*** Cervicitis Flow length decrease Moniliasis ***PROGESTIN DEFICIENCY*** Breakthrough bleeding and spotting during pill days 10 to 21 Delayed withdrawal bleeding Dysmenorrhea (also estrogen excess) Heavy flow and clots (also es- trogen excess), hyper-men- orrhea, menorrhagia	***ESTROGEN EXCESS OR PROGESTERONE DEFICIENCY*** Bloating Dizziness, syncope Edema Headache (cyclic) Irritability Leg cramps Nausea, vomiting Visual changes (cyclic) Weight gain (cyclic)

III. GENERAL		IV. CARDIOVASCULAR SYSTEM
ESTROGEN EXCESS Chloasma Chronic nasal pharyngitis Gastric influenza and varicella Hay fever and allergic rhinitis Urinary tract infection *ESTROGEN DEFICIENCY* Nervousness Vasomotor symptoms	*PROGESTIN EXCESS* Appetite increase Depression Fatigue Hypoglycemia symptoms Libido decrease Neurodermatitis Weight gain (non-cyclic) *ANDROGEN EXCESS* Acne Cholestatic jaundice Hirsutism Libido increase Oily skin and scalp Rash and pruritus Edema	*PROGESTIN EXCESS* Hypertension Leg vein dilation *ESTROGEN EXCESS* Capillary fragility Cerebrovascular accident Deep vein thrombosis hemi- paresis (unilateral weakness and numbness) Telangiectasias Thromboembolic disease

TABLE 12 – Symptoms of a Serious or Potentially Serious Nature

SYMPTOM	POSSIBLE CAUSE
SERIOUS: Pills should be stopped immediately.	
Loss of vision, proptosis, diplopia, papilledema	Retinal artery thrombosis
Unilateral numbness, weakness or tingling	Hemorrhagic or thrombotic stroke
Severe pains in chest, left arm or neck	Myocardial infarction
Hemoptysis	Pulmonary embolism
Severe pains, tenderness or swelling, warmth or palpable cord in legs	Thrombophlebitis
Slurring of speech	Hemorrhagic or thrombotic stroke
Hepatic mass or tenderness	Liver neoplasm

POTENTIALLY SERIOUS: Pills may be continued with caution while patient is being evaluated.	
Absence of menses	Pregnancy
Spotting or breakthrough bleeding	Cervical, endometrial or vaginal cancer
Breast mass, pain or swelling	Breast cancer
Right upper-quadrant pain	Cholecystitis, cholelithiasis or liver neoplasm
Mid-epigastric pain	Thrombosis of abdominal artery or vein, myocardial infarction or pulmonary embolism
Migraine (vascular or throbbing) headache	Vascular spasm which may precede thrombosis
Severe nonvascular headache	Hypertension, vascular spasm
Galactorrhea	Pituitary adenoma
Jaundice, pruritus	Cholestatic jaundice
Depression	B_6 deficiency
Uterine size increase	Leiomyomata, adenomyosis, pregnancy

TABLE 13 – Vitamin and Mineral Changes Associated with Oral Contraceptives

NUTRIENT	SERUM PLASMA OR BLOOD LEVEL CHANGES	EARLY CLINICAL EFFECTS	MINIMUM DAILY REQUIREMENTS ADULTS	BEST DIETARY SOURCES
Vitamin A	Increased	Fissured skin, coarsening of hair, hepatomegaly	4,000 to 5,000 IU	Liver, kidney, dairy products, eggs
Thiamine (B_1)	Decreased	Anorexia, lethargy, depression, irritability (beriberi)	1 mg	Pork, wheat germ
Riboflavin (B_2)	Decreased	Glossitis, seborrhea, fissures of the corners of the mouth, conjunctival irritation	1.2 mg	Milk, cheese
Pyridoxine (B_6)	Decreased	Clinical depression, glucose intolerance	2.0 mg	Yeast, wheat germ, meat, bananas
Cobalamin (B_{12})	Decreased	Potentiates pernicious anemia, folacin deficiency	3 mcg	Liver, kidney, fresh milk

Ascorbic acid (C)	Decreased	Bleeding gums, swollen, tender joints (scurvy)	45 mg	Citrus fruits, raw vegetables, tomatoes
Folacin (folic acid)	Decreased	Megaloblastic anemia, gastrointestinal disturbances	0.4 mg	Liver, kidney beans, lima beans, green leafy vegetables
Calcium	Decreased	None	1 gm	Milk, cheese
Copper	Increased	Pigment changes, Wilson's disease (hepatolenticular degeneration)	2 mg	Liver, shellfish, whole grains, cherries
Iron	Increased	None	10 mg	Liver, meat, egg yolk, green leafy vegetables
Magnesium	Decreased	Weight loss, change in hair, depression, muscle weakness	350 mg	Whole grain cereals, nuts, meats, milk
Zinc	Decreased	Delayed wound healing, alopecia, loss of taste	15 mg	Meat, liver, eggs, seafood

TABLE 14 – Drugs That May Affect Oral Contraceptive Activities

CLASS OF COMPOUND	DRUG	PROPOSED METHOD OF ACTION	SUGGESTED MANAGEMENT	REF.
Anticonvulsant Drugs	Barbiturates: Phenobarbital Primidone Hydantoins: Phenytoin Mephenytoin Ethotoin Succinimide: Ethosuximide Carbamazepine	Induction of liver microsomal enzymes; rapid metabolism of estrogen and increased binding of progestin and ethinyl estradiol to sex hormone binding globulin.	Use another method, another drug or higher dose OC (50 mcg ethinyl estradiol)	14 70 268 297
Cholesterol Lowering Agent	Clofibrate	Reduces elevated serum triglycerides and cholesterol	Use another method	322 13 15
Antituberculosis Antibiotics and Antifungals	Rifampin Penicillin Ampicillin Cotrimoxazole Griseofulvin Minocycline	Rifampin increases metabolism of progestins Enterohepatic circulation disturbance, intestinal hurry	For short course, use additional method or use another drug	124 199 375

Antituberculosis Antibiotics and Antifungals	Metronidazole Tetracycline Neomycin Chloramphenicol Sulfonamide Nitrofurantoin	Induction of microsomal liver enzymes; see above	For long course, use another method	198 268
Sedatives and Hypnotics	Benzodiazepines Chloral hydrate Antimigraine preparations	Increased microsomal liver enzymes; see above	For short course, use additional method or another drug For long course, use another method or higher dose OCs	268

Drugs That May Increase Oral Contraceptive Steroid Activities

Antipyretics	Acetaminophen	Reduces sulphation of ethinyl estradiol in the gut	None needed unless symptoms of excess estrogen occur	375

TABLE 15 — Modification of Other Drug Activity by Oral Contraceptives

CLASS OF COMPOUND	DRUG	MODIFICATION OF DRUG ACTION	SUGGESTED MANAGEMENT	REF.
Antibiotics	Troleandomycin Cyclosporine	Increased serum levels and possible liver damage	Do not use OC with these antibiotics	124 375
Anticoagulants	All	OCs increase clotting factors, decrease efficacy	Do not use OC with anticoagulant	24 268
Anticonvulsants	All	Fluid retention, increases seizures	Use another method	14 70 154
Antidiabetic agents	Insulin and oral hypoglycemic agents	High dose OCs cause impaired glucose tolerance	Use low dose estrogen and progestin OC or use another method	78 268 418
Antihypertensive agents	Guanethidine methyldopa	Estrogen component causes Na retention; progestin has no effect	Use low estrogen OC or another method Possible need for dosage increase	268 474

Alpha-II adrenoreceptor agents	Clonidine	Increases sedation effect	Use with caution	12 34
Antipyretics and analgesics	Acetaminophen Aspirin Morphine	Increased renal clearance	Increased dose may be necessary	
	Antipyrine Meperidine	Impaired metabolism	Decrease dosage	207
Benzodiazepines	Chlordiazepoxide Lorazepam Oxazepam Diazepam Nitrazepam Alprazolam Triazolam Temazepam	Increases effects, decreases clearance or increased metabolism	Use with caution	88 268 375
Beta-blocking agents	Metoprolol Oxprenolol Propanolol	Increases drug effect	Decrease dosage if necessary	121 268 375

Continued ➡

TABLE 15 — Modification of Other Drug Activity by Oral Contraceptives (continued)

CLASS OF COMPOUND	DRUG	MODIFICATION OF DRUG ACTION	SUGGESTED MANAGEMENT	REF.
Betamimetics	Isoproterenol agents	Estrogen causes decreased response to these drugs	Adjust dose of drug as necessary. Discontinuing OCs can result in excessive drug activity	109 121
Bronchodilators	All	Decreases oxidation, leading to possible toxicity	Use with caution	459
Cholesterol-lowering agents	Clofibrate	Increased clearance rate	Increase dose	375
Corticosteroids	Prednisone Prednisolone	Markedly increases serum levels	Possible need for dosage decrease	459 375
Dopamine agonists	Apomorphine	Decreased effect	Higher dose may be necessary	375
Methylxanthines	Caffeine Theophylline Methylxanthine	Higher serum levels due to decreased clearance	Use with caution	375

| Phenothiazine tranquilizers | All phenothiazines, reserpine, and similar drugs | Estrogen potentiates the hyperprolactinemia effect of these drugs | Use other drugs or lower dose OCs. If galactorrhea or hyperprolactinemia occurs, use another method | 88 |
| Tricyclic antidepressants | Clomipramine Imipramine Amitriptyline | Increased serum levels due to decreased clearance | Decrease dosage or use another method | 154 375 |

TABLE 16 – Cardiovascular Disease Mortality in Oral Contraceptive Users,
Former Users and Controls

	MORTALITY RATE PER 100,000 WOMEN/YEARS				
CAUSE	CURRENT USERS	FORMER USERS	CONTROLS	CURRENT USERS vs. CONTROLS	FORMER USERS vs. CONTROLS
All nonrheumatic heart disease and hypertension	15.1	9.6	2.1	7.3	4.6
Ischemic heart disease	13.0	4.1	2.0	6.4	2.0
Malignant hypertension	0.0	2.5	0.0	–	–
All cerebrovascular disease	10.1	18.2	5.0	2.0	3.6
Subarachnoid hemorrhage	7.3	10.2	2.3	3.2	4.5
Cerebral thrombosis, hemorrhage and embolism	2.7	8.1	2.7	1.0	3.0
Pulmonary embolism and thrombophlebitis	2.8	2.2	0.0	–	–
Other vascular diseases	0.8	0.9	0.0	–	–
All circulatory diseases	28.6	30.9	7.2	4.0	4.3

Reference: 359

TABLE 17 – Circulatory Mortality by Age, Smoking Status, and Oral Contraceptive Use

| | MORTALITY RATE PER 100,000 WOMEN/YEARS | | USERS vs. CONTROLS | |
	EVER-USERS	CONTROLS	RELATIVE RISK	EXCESS DEATHS
AGE 15 to 24				
Nonsmokers	0.0	0.0	–	0.0
Smokers	10.5	0.0	–	10.5
AGE 25 to 34				
Nonsmokers	4.4	2.7	1.6	1.7
Smokers	14.2	4.2	3.4	10.0
AGE 35 to 44				
Nonsmokers	21.5	6.4	3.3	15.1
Smokers	63.4	15.2	4.2	48.2
AGE 45+				
Nonsmokers	52.4	11.4	4.6	40.9
Smokers	206.7	27.9	7.4	178.8
All Women	29.9	7.2	4.2	22.7

Reference: 359

General Information	Patient Complaints/ Cross References
	Starting OCs
	Stopping OCs
	Initial Selection of OCs
	Implanted Contraceptives
	Injected Contraceptives
	Emergency Contraception
	Other Hormonal and Developmental Contraceptives
Reproductive System Side Effects	Uterine Changes/Ovarian Changes
	Breast Disorders
	Post Pill Amenorrhea/Galactorrhea
Other Systemic Effects	Nutritional and Weight Changes
	Musculosketetal System
	Neuropsychological System
	Neurosensory System
	Respiratory/Urinary Systems
Index	Index/Abbreviations

#18 Patient Complaints/Cross References

The following list contains common patient complaints that may be due to side effects occurring because of OC use (also see Tables 11 and 12). Many OC users experience no side effects, and many health problems have no relation to OC use. However, since these symptoms could possibly be caused or aggravated by OC use, they are included in this listing, followed by the section number(s) where information concerning this symptom can be found:

Symptom   **Tab Section #**

18.

Symptom	Tab Section #

#19 Starting OCs

General Information

Physical Examination and Follow-Up
A complete medical history and physical examination [see Section #21] should be taken prior to the initiation or reinstitution of oral contraceptives and at least annually during use of oral contraceptives. These physical examinations should include special reference to blood pressure, breasts, abdomen and pelvic organs, including cervical cytology and relevant laboratory tests. In case of undiagnosed, persistent, or recurrent abnormal vaginal bleeding, appropriate diagnostic measures should be conducted to rule out malignancy. Women with a strong family history of breast cancer or who have breast nodules should be monitored with particular care.

-FDA Package Insert Labeling

OCs should be prescribed for no more than one year until a follow-up physical examination is performed.

Patients are most likely to forget or skip pills during the first cycles of use. It is important to instruct new OC starters about what to do if they miss taking their pills. A 1997 study found that 48 percent of patients skipped two or more pills in a row at least once during the first three months of use (Ref 295). Of these, 27 percent did not use a backup method or abstain from intercourse after missing two or more pills. Patients were more likely to miss pills if they were single, did not have strong support from their partners, or had sex frequently.

Instructions about Early Side Effects

Some side effects are common during the first through the third cycles of OC use, but these should disappear spontaneously thereafter. These side effects include breakthrough bleeding (BTB) and spotting (see Section #9) and symptoms associated with early pregnancy, especially nausea.

Patients should be encouraged to wait until the third cycle of OC use before seeking a change in or considering discontinuing OCs unless the side effect is one of those associated with serious disease.

Patients should be informed about symptoms of potentially serious side effects and warned to discontinue OCs and seek medical assistance at once if such symptoms occur (Tables 11 and 12).

Onset of Effectiveness

Prevention of ovulation may not occur if OCs are started after the fifth menstrual cycle day. Although other contraceptive actions (such as changes in the cervix, uterus, or endometrium) may occur, 48 to 72 hours may be required before these changes are sufficient to prevent conception.

OCs should be started on the first menstrual cycle day or on a Sunday. If started on a Sunday, the patient should take her first tablet on the first Sunday after her menstrual period begins. If her period begins on a Sunday, she should take the first tablet on that same day. A backup method, such as condoms or foam, should be used for the first seven days in initial cycles.

After the first cycle, OCs should be restarted no later than seven days after the last progestin-containing OC has been taken. Other recommendations, such as to wait until the onset of menses and then count five more days before restarting active OCs, are no longer valid for low-dose OCs and may result in pregnancy.

The synthetic steroids in OCs are not completely eliminated from the body within 24 hours; therefore, their effect is cumulative, with a buildup over several days. Maximum effectiveness may not be reached until after seven days.

If progestin-only or very low-dose OCs are used or if combination OCs are started after the fifth day post menstruation, **additional contraceptive methods for the first seven days of OC use will assure maximum effectiveness**.

OC effectiveness may also be correlated with patient compliance. Patients not accustomed to taking daily pills may need to be counseled to use backup contraception during the first cycle or until pill-taking becomes habitual.

Forgotten or Missed Tablets

Patients will occasionally forget to take tablets. To help them remember to take their pills so that maximum effectiveness may be achieved, clinicians should emphasize that patients take their OCs at the same time each day.

It is important that patients also be instructed what to do if they forget to take one or more OCs. Patients should be instructed to use additional contraceptive measures for the rest of their cycles if they forget to take two or more pills. Additionally, they should be advised to follow the procedures listed in the following chart.

Consecutive OCs Omitted	Time in Cycle	Instructions to Patients*
1	Anytime	Take missed OC immediately and next OC at regular time
2	First two weeks	Take two OCs daily for next two days; then resume taking OCs on regular schedule. Use barrier contraception for the remainder of the cycle
2	Third week	Take one OC daily until last day; dispose of remaining OCs; begin new OC cycle that same day
3 or more	Anytime	Take one OC daily until last day; dispose of remaining OCs; begin new OC cycle that same day

*Additional contraceptive measures should be started immediately as soon as the omission of OCs is discovered. These additional measures should be used for at least seven days.

If menstruation does not occur at the regular time, a pregnancy test must be performed. If menstruation does occur, OCs should be restarted either five days after the onset of menstruation (as for the first cycle of OCs) or seven days after the last active tablet, whichever is earlier. Patients should be instructed to use additional contraceptive measures throughout the cycle if they stop and restart OCs.

Special Instructions for OC Use
Some patients need special instructions when starting OCs. Included in this group are those patients who:
- Recently delivered after full-term pregnancy
- Are nursing
- Recently had a spontaneous or induced abortion
- Have infrequent or irregular cycles
- Are taking other medications

Postpartum Thromboembolism
Since the immediate postpartum period . . . is associated with an increased risk of thromboembolism, oral contraceptives should be started no earlier than four to six weeks after delivery in women who elect not to breastfeed.

-FDA Package Insert Labeling

Recent Pregnancy
Because of the increased incidence of spontaneous thromboembolism following delivery, some experts recommend that combination OCs not be started until the third postpartum week. If the patient is not nursing, she may start combination OCs three to four weeks postpartum without waiting for her first menstrual cycle.

Ovulation rarely occurs before the fourth week following a full-term delivery. If OCs are started at this time, the incidence of BTB is low and patients are not likely to become pregnant if the first menses is delayed. However, if prolactin-suppressing drugs (such as bromocriptine [Parlodel®, Sandoz]) are used to suppress lactation, ovulation may occur earlier and OCs should be started by the 14th postpartum day. Because they are not associated with an increased risk of thromboembolism, progestin-only pills may be started immediately postpartum unless the new mother is nursing (see Section #7).

Nursing

Steroid components of OCs may be found in the breastmilk of nursing mothers. Additionally, combination OCs may inhibit lactation. For these reasons, many physicians recommend that nursing mothers not start OCs until their infants are weaned. Any OCs used during nursing should contain very low doses of estrogen and progestin so that milk production is not inhibited and the amount of drug in the breastmilk is minimized. (See Section #7 for additional information.)

Recent Abortion

Because OCs reduce risks of thromboembolism and because of the possibility of ovulation within 14 days following spontaneous or induced abortion, OCs should be started immediately or, at the latest, within seven days following a first-trimester abortion (five to 13 weeks). Following a mid-trimester abortion, OCs should be started in the same manner as following a full-term pregnancy (see Section #7).

Irregular Menstrual Cycles

Women with amenorrhea or infrequent or irregular menstrual cycles may start OCs at any time if they are not pregnant and no other contraindications exist. Additional contraceptive methods should be used for the first cycle.

Women with irregular cycles may remain anovulatory or become amenorrheic after discontinuing OCs if they have histories of:

- Oligomenorrhea
- Secondary amenorrhea
- Irregular menstrual cycles

Women with these pre-existing problems should be advised of the possibility of amenorrhea and encouraged to use other contraceptive methods. Amenorrhea and anovulatory cycles may also occur in women who have not previously experienced menstrual irregularities.

Concurrent Drug Therapy

Contraceptive effectiveness may lessen and BTB and spotting may occur when OCs are taken concurrently with medications used for certain medical conditions (see Table 14 for a complete list), including:

- Insomnia or nervous disorders - Barbiturates
- Fungal infections (e.g., ringworm) - Griseofulvin
- Epilepsy - Phenytoin, ethotoin, mephenytoin

Patients taking these medications should use additional contraception during all OC cycles or use a different contraceptive method.

References: 8, 83, 109, 110, 198, 228, 295, 329, 436

#20 Stopping OCs

General Information
Reasons for Stopping OCs
Resumption of Menses After OC Use

GENERAL INFORMATION

Reasons for discontinuing OCs include:
- Side effects
- Missed menses
- Length of use
- Age of user
- Surgery and/or hospitalization involving increased risk of thromboembolism
- Desire for pregnancy

A delay in the resumption of normal menstrual cycles or in conception may occur after OCs are discontinued. It is recommended that patients delay conception for one to three months after discontinuing OC use.

When OCs are discontinued before reproductive capacity has ended, other highly effective methods of birth control, such as IUDs or surgical sterilization, are often recommended. Barrier methods, e.g., diaphragms, condoms, and spermicidal agents, are less effective. Estimated pregnancy rates per year for barrier methods are:
- 9.2 for ages 35 to 39
- 3.4 for ages 40 to 44

REASONS FOR STOPPING OCs

Side Effects

OCs should be stopped immediately whenever potentially dangerous side effects occur (Table 12). Other contraceptive means should be selected for these patients, since the risks associated with pregnancy are usually greater than those associated with OC use.

If OCs are stopped prior to the tenth day of use, menstruation may not occur; if it does occur, it may be prolonged. OCs should be taken for at least the first 10 days of the cycle if it is safe and feasible for the patient to do so.

Absence of Menses

20

It is recommended that for any patient who has missed two consecutive periods, pregnancy should be ruled out before continuing oral contraceptive use. If the patient has not adhered to the prescribed schedule, the possibility should be considered at the time of the first missed period. Oral contraceptive use should be discontinued if pregnancy is confirmed.

-FDA Package Insert Labeling

Clinical Information

If a patient has not strictly adhered to her prescribed OC regimen (especially if progestin-only OCs are used), clinicians should consider the possibility of pregnancy for patients whose menses have not occurred after the first cycle of OCs or after 45 days from their last menstrual periods. OCs should be withheld until pregnancy has been ruled out.

Patients can become pregnant even if they have adhered to their prescribed OC regimens.

Causal Factors

The most common cause for absence of menses while taking OCs is lack of endometrial stimulation due to low estrogenic activity (see Section #9). Absence of menses because of low estrogenic activity is often accompanied by spotting or breakthrough bleeding (BTB) during the days when OCs are taken.

Management

A pregnancy test should be performed as a first step. Absence of menses is not harmful and most often occurs in the first cycles of OC use, although it may also occur after OCs have been used for many months because of endometrial atrophy. If lack of menses is due to low estrogenic activity, a pelvic examination will usually reveal the uterus to be smaller than normal size. If a pregnancy test is negative, the dose of OCs should be adjusted and the regimen continued. Generally, OCs with the lowest incidence of BTB and spotting also have the lowest incidence of absence of menses. Other methods of contraception should be used if OCs are discontinued.

Length of OC Use

The most recent studies have shown that the length of OC use is not a major factor in the development of serious side effects, as long as the patient's age is within acceptable limits. There is no need to stop OCs because of length of use.

Age of OC User

Estimates of Mortality from Contraceptive Use

. . . The observation of a possible increase in risk of mortality with age for oral contraceptive users is based on data gathered in the 1970s, but not reported in the U.S. until 1983. However, current clinical practice involves the use of lower estrogen dose formulations combined with careful restriction of oral contraceptive use to women who do not have the various risk factors listed in this labeling.

Because of these changes in practice and also because of some limited new data which suggest that the risk of cardiovascular disease with the use of oral contraceptives may now be less than previously observed, the Fertility and Maternal Health Drugs Advisory Committee was asked to review the topic in 1989. The Committee concluded that, although cardiovascular disease risks may be increased with oral contraceptive use after age 40 in healthy non-smoking women (even with the newer low-dose formulations), there are greater potential health risks associated with pregnancy in older women and with the alternative surgical and medical problems which may be necessary if such women do not have access to effective and acceptable means of contraception.

Therefore, the Committee recommended that the benefits of oral contraceptive use by healthy non-smoking women over 40 may outweigh the possible risks. Of course, older women, as well as all women who take oral contraceptives, should take the lowest possible dose formulation that is effective.

-FDA Package Insert Labeling

OCs are as safe as other conventional contraceptive methods (which may fail and result in pregnancy) for women up to age 45 who do not smoke and for women up to age 35 who do. When OCs first became available, no age limit was recommended and OCs were often taken until the fifth decade. Since that time, a large body of evidence has shown that women who use OCs are at increased risk of developing cardiovascular disease (CVD) as they get older, especially if they smoke cigarettes.

In 1977 the Royal College of Obstetrics and Gynecology (RCOG) and the Royal College of General Practitioners (RCGP) recommended that women older than age 35 should discontinue OC use. In 1981, the RCGP changed its recommendation to state that women who do not smoke may take OCs until age 45 and that women who smoke should stop OCs at age 35.

In 1990, the FDA instructed manufacturers to revise OC labels to reflect the current scientific opinion that the benefits of OC use for healthy, nonsmokers older than age 40 may outweigh possible risks. To minimize risks, older women should be cautioned to take the lowest dose combination formulation that is effective (Ref 6).

Table 17 shows the excess risk for each age group for smokers and nonsmokers.

Surgery and/or Hospitalization

Pre- and Postoperative Thromboembolism

A two- to six-fold increase in relative risk of postoperative thromboembolic complications has been reported with the use of oral contraceptives. If feasible, oral contraceptives should be discontinued at least four weeks prior to and for two weeks after elective surgery and during and following prolonged immobilization. Since the immediate postpartum period also is associated with an increased risk of thromboembolism, oral contraceptives should be started no earlier than four to six weeks after delivery in women who elect not to breastfeed.

-FDA Package Insert Labeling

OCs should be stopped prior to elective surgery requiring hospitalization or immobilization of an extremity because of the increased risk of venous thromboembolism (VTE). A four- to sixfold increased risk of postsurgery VTE has been reported in OC users. Although the exact length of time necessary to avoid this risk is not known, OCs should be discontinued for at least four weeks before surgery or prolonged immobilization. Stopping OCs for shorter periods may also be helpful. Progestin-only OCs need not be discontinued.

Other methods of birth control should be substituted for OCs if continued contraception is needed or desired during this period. OCs may be resumed after the period of bed rest or immobilization has ended. When OCs are resumed, the same directions should be followed as for initially starting OCs (see Section #19).

Wound healing has been reported to be disturbed following tooth extractions in OC patients.

References: 109, 110, 130, 330, 331, 359, 457, 459, 469

RESUMPTION OF MENSES AFTER OC USE

Patients may experience a delay in resumption of normal menstruation after discontinuing OCs. For women whose cycles were regular before OC use, the delay will be brief and the first menstrual period should occur by the fifth week after the last tablet is taken. Those who had irregular or infrequent menses (oligomenorrhea) before taking OCs may have a delay of three months or longer before resuming their previous menstrual pattern. Some patients with previous irregular menses will have one or more regular menstrual cycles before resuming their former patterns.

Failure to have the first menses within three months may be the result of:
- Pregnancy
- Post-pill amenorrhea (see Section #28)
- Menopause

All possibilities should be considered. Meanwhile, patients who do not wish to become pregnant should use other contraceptive methods.

It is important for physicians to inform patients who discontinue OC use that the absence of menses does not necessarily indicate pregnancy and that they should not stop using other contraceptive methods until pregnancy is confirmed by an appropriate test.

Menopause will cause some pregnancy tests to be positive. Older patients should be informed of this possibility.

References: 8, 84, 162, 291, 356, 439, 440

NOTES

#21 Initial Selection of OCs

Criteria for Choice of OC
Contraindications
Steroid Dose
Patient Characteristics
Menstrual Characteristics
Hormone Sensitivity

CRITERIA FOR CHOICE OF OC

> All women who take oral contraceptives should take the lowest possible dose formulation that is effective.
>
> *-FDA Package Insert Labeling*

Factors that should be considered in choosing an OC are:
- Physical examination and laboratory findings
- Contraindications
- Steroid dose
- Patient's personal/family health characteristics
- Patient's menstrual characteristics
- Patient's hormone sensitivity

Initial Examination Findings
The initial physical and laboratory examinations should result in normal findings in:
- Blood pressure
- Breasts
- Liver palpation
- Pelvic examination
- Thyroid palpation
- Extremities
- Papanicolaou (Pap) smear
- Cholesterol (for women ages 40 and older who have family histories of heart disease), including:
  - Total
  - High-density lipoprotein (HDL)
  - Low-density lipoprotein (LDL)
- Triglycerides (for women ages 40 and older who have family histories of heart disease)

- Fasting blood sugar (for women who have family histories of nonrheumatic heart disease or diabetes)
- Leiden factor V (for patients who have personal or family histories of venous thromboembolism [VTE])

CONTRAINDICATIONS

Absolute Contraindications

Oral contraceptives should not be used in women who have the following conditions:
- Thrombophlebitis/thromboembolic disorders
- A past history of deep vein thrombophlebitis or thromboembolic disorders
- Cerebral vascular or coronary artery disease
- Known or suspected carcinoma of the breast
- Known or suspected carcinoma of the endometrium and known or suspected estrogen-dependent neoplasia
- Undiagnosed abnormal genital bleeding
- Cholestatic jaundice of pregnancy or jaundice with prior pill use
- Hepatic adenomas, carcinomas, or benign liver tumors
- Known or suspected pregnancy (see Section #7)

-FDA Package Insert Labeling

21

Other absolute contraindications are:
- Markedly impaired liver function
- Benign or malignant liver tumor that developed during previous use of OCs or other estrogen-containing products
- Type II hyperlipidemia (hypercholesterolemia)
- Leiden factor V mutation

Relative Contraindications

Relative contraindications to OC use are:
- Migraine or vascular headache
- Cardiac or renal dysfunction
- Gestational diabetes or impaired glucose tolerance
- Diastolic blood pressure of 90 mm Hg or greater or hypertension by any other criteria
- Psychic depression
- Varicose veins
- Ages 35 and older for smokers*

- Sickle-cell or sickle cell-hemoglobin C disease
- Cholestatic jaundice during pregnancy
- Worsening of any chronic condition during pregnancy
- Hepatitis or mononucleosis during past year
- Nursing
- Asthma
- First-order family histories of nonrheumatic cardiovascular disease (CVD) or diabetes before age 50
- Use of drugs known to interact with OCs
- Ulcerative colitis

*Some physicians consider smoking after age 35 as an absolute contraindication.

References: 97, 109, 110, 330, 331

STEROID DOSE

Amount

Ideally, OCs should contain 35 mcg or less ethinyl estradiol (EE) and the equivalent of 0.4 or 0.5 mg norethindrone. OCs with estrogen doses above 35 mcg may increase the incidence of thromboembolic disease. Progestins at doses as low as 1.0 mg norethindrone, 0.3 mg norgestrel, or 0.15 mg levonorgestrel (LNG) can cause significant changes in serum lipid and insulin levels, which may result in atherosclerotic vascular changes (Tables 6 and 7 and see Section #12).

Short- vs Long-Term Use

For short-term therapeutic use and as an aid in decreasing initial breakthrough bleeding (BTB) and spotting, OCs containing more than 35 mcg estrogen and progestins with activities greater than 0.5 mg norethindrone may be prescribed. After initial cycles and for continued long-term use, OCs containing 35 mcg or less estrogen and progestin with progestational and androgenic activities equal to 0.5 mg or less norethindrone should be selected.

Multiphasic OCs in which estrogen and progestin doses are variable should contain total amounts of estrogen and progestin that do not exceed those of recommended combination OCs given for 21 days.

Increasing the dose of estrogen may reduce the adverse effect of progestin on serum lipid levels to some degree, but the risk of thromboembolic disease due to estrogens may be increased to an even greater extent.

The appropriate dose and type of progestin significantly reduce the adverse effects of OCs on many metabolic markers of risk for coronary artery disease. Progestin-only formulations or combinations containing desogestrel or low-dose norethindrone were associated with the most favorable profiles.

OCs that meet the presently recommended criteria for safe long-term use (e.g., that have no adverse effects on serum lipids or clotting factors) are listed in Groups 1, 2, 5, 7, and 8 of Table 9.

Doses of other progestins that result in activities equivalent to 0.4 or 0.5 mg norethindrone (Table 3) are:

- For progestational activity:
  - 0.05 mg gestodene
  - 0.06 mg desogestrel
  - 0.1 mg levonorgestrel (LNG)
  - 0.2 mg dl-norgestrel
  - 0.36 mg ethynodiol diacetate
  - 0.4 mg norgestimate
  - 0.43 mg norethindrone acetate
- For androgenic activity:
  - 0.05 mg levonorgestrel (LNG)
  - 0.1 mg dl-norgestrel
  - 0.15 mg desogestrel
  - 0.05 mg gestodene
  - 0.2 mg norgestimate
  - 0.3 mg norethindrone acetate
  - 0.8 mg ethynodiol diacetate

References: 89, 111, 137, 187, 404, 441

PATIENT CHARACTERISTICS

Predisposing Factors to CVD

An increased risk of myocardial infarction (MI) and cerebrovascular accident (CVA) in OC users and nonusers is associated with the following factors:

- Type II hyperlipidemia (hypercholesterolemia)
- Diabetes mellitus
- Hypertension
- Previous hypertension in pregnancy
- Obesity
- Smoking (see Section #12, *Myocardial Infarction*)
- Leiden factor V mutation

The effect of these factors for MI is synergistic, and the risk is multiplied with an increase in the number of factors:

- One factor - Four times increased risk
- Two factors - 10 times increased risk
- Three factors - 78 times increased risk

An increased risk of venous thromboembolism (VTE) is associated with:

- Obesity
- Varicose veins of the lower extremities
- Immobilization of a limb or of the entire body because of illness
- History of previous VTE

Women who experienced thrombophlebitis during pregnancy or when not taking OCs are particularly likely to have such occurrences when taking OCs.

References: 109, 110, 330, 331

Family History of CVD and Diabetes

A history of nonrheumatic CVD or diabetes before age 50 in first-order relatives indicates a possible hereditary factor. OCs should not be used in most such cases. In some circumstances, OCs may be used if:

- Blood cholesterol levels are below 267 mg per 100 ml

- Triglyceride levels are below 207 mg per 100 ml
- Consideration is given to:
  - The relative's age at the time of the onset of CVD
  - Underlying factors that may have affected onset of CVD

Patients with actual diabetes need effective contraception. OCs with low, balanced doses of estrogen and low progestational activities should be chosen.

Persistence of Risk
Formerly, the risk of dying from CVD was four times higher in OC users than nonusers and remained increased to the same degree in former OC users for an unknown number of years after OCs are discontinued (Table 16). There now appears to be no long-term risk following use of sub-50 mcg estrogen OCs. However, this may only be true if the OCs contain low doses of progestins, which do not have adverse effects on serum lipids (see Tables 6 and 7).

References: 26, 186, 252, 253, 254, 255, 256, 355, 357, 359, 454, 469, 499

Age and OC Use
The risk of CVD increases progressively after age 30. However, continued OC use is safer than pregnancy in women up to age 35 who smoke and in women of all ages who do not.

For women younger than age 18, there is no reason not to prescribe OCs for:
- Contraception
- Regulation on menses
- Treatment of menstrual-related symptoms
- Other medical indications

There is no evidence of a harmful effect of OCs on the reproductive health of women younger than age 18 who have experienced menstrual cycles for at least 12 months. To the contrary, there is considerable evidence that endometriosis and pelvic infections, two common causes of infertility and disability, are less severe or occur less frequently in young women who use OCs.

During the first year or two of menstruation, cycles are often irregular and anovulatory; symptoms of androgen excess (acne) frequently occur at this time. OCs have been used to treat acne in these patients without harmful effects.

Height growth usually ceases within one year of the first menses. Administration of sex steroids after menstruation starts does not appear to alter the final height attained.

References: 26, 252, 255

Weight and OC Use

Underweight women are more likely to experience side effects of hormone excess, such as:
- Nausea
- Vomiting
- Breast discomfort
- Cramps
- Weight gain

However, underweight women have less BTB and spotting than over- and normal-weight women and react most favorably to OCs with low estrogen doses and low progestational activities.

Overweight women usually have more BTB and spotting during first cycles of OC use, but compared to normal to underweight women, they have:
- Fewer minor side effects
- Less weight gain
- Less change in diastolic pressure

Overweight women may need OCs with higher endometrial activities initially.

MENSTRUAL CHARACTERISTICS

Clinical Information

The major reason for patient dissatisfaction and discontinuance of OCs is menstrual irregularity, including such characteristics as:

- BTB
- Spotting
- Failure of withdrawal menses

Bleeding irregularity is greatest during the first cycle of OC use and thereafter decreases until a plateau is reached in the third or fourth cycle. Bleeding irregularity rarely improves after the fourth cycle and may worsen. OCs that have high endometrial activities may be used during these early cycles to encourage continuation of use in new patients. However, in order to achieve the maximum possible menstrual control, there is no need to exceed limits of 50 mcg EE.

After the initial cycles, all OC patients should be switched to formulations with sub-50 mcg estrogen doses and low or intermediate androgenic activities for continued long-term use (Table 9, Groups 2 and 4-9). For initial cycles, however, side effects may be reduced if OCs are selected on the basis of a patient's menstrual pattern and history of sex steroid-related symptoms. These factors provide a good general indication of the level of endometrial activity the patient will initially require in order to maintain satisfactory cycles (Table 8). However, choosing an OC merely to avoid one specific side effect may result in the occurrence of other side effects.

Menstrual Types

OCs can be chosen on the basis of the following menstrual types:

- LIGHT FLOW AND MILD CRAMPS - Women with two to four days of light flow and mild or no cramps react favorably to OCs with low endometrial activities during all cycles

- MODERATE FLOW AND AVERAGE CRAMPS - Women with four to six days of flow and average cramps may require OCs with slightly stronger endometrial activities during initial cycles. Low endometrial activity OCs may be used if initial-cycle BTB and spotting are acceptable to the patient
- HEAVY FLOW AND SEVERE CRAMPS - Women with six to seven days of flow or longer and severe cramps require initial OCs with higher endometrial activities. In addition to requiring increased progestin doses or progestational activities, these women may also require more estrogen (50 mcg) to balance the increased progestational activity. Before a high progestin dose is chosen (1 mg norethindrone equivalent or greater), patients should be examined for a predisposition to hypertension
- IRREGULAR MENSES - Women with infrequent or irregular menses are often anovulatory. Such patients often have polycystic ovaries (sclerocystic ovaries, Stein-Leventhal syndrome) when anovulatory cycles are associated with:
  - Heavy flow
  - Acne, increased sebum, or hirsutism (see Section #15)
  - Obesity

OCs with low androgenic but high progestational activities may be needed to suppress endogenous ovarian androgen production.

Irregular menses with excess androgen effects may be caused by:
- Ovarian tumors
- Adrenal tumors
- Adrenal hyperplasia
- Stromal hyperplasia
- Enzyme defects

Irregular cycles and amenorrhea without androgen effects may be associated with:
- Normal or abnormal pregnancy
- Hypothalamic insufficiency

- Pituitary tumor
- Ovarian failure
- Endometriosis
- Pelvic inflammatory disease (PID)
- Diabetes
- Hypothyroidism
- Other medical diseases

OCs should not be given to patients with irregular cycles until appropriate tests have been conducted.

Patients with infrequent or irregular cycles should be advised that they are likely to return to their former menstrual patterns when OCs are discontinued and that OCs may hide the progressive worsening of menstrual irregularity (see Sections #9, #10, and #28).

References: 81, 83, 87

HORMONE SENSITIVITY

Clinical Information
Some women demonstrate increased or decreased sensitivity to their own natural sex hormones. Evidence of this sensitivity may have occurred during periods of physiological hormone excess, such as pregnancy, or at the time of low hormone levels preceding or during menses.

Estrogen-Sensitive Women
Symptoms of excessive sensitivity to estrogen or of elevated estrogen levels include:
- Unusually severe nausea or edema during pregnancy or at menstrual midcycle
- Enlarged uterus
- Uterine fibroids
- Cervical hypertrophy
- Large breasts
- Fibrocystic disease of the breast
- Heavy menstruation
- Severe cramps during menstruation

Low estrogenic activity OCs should be chosen initially for these patients.

Progesterone-Sensitive Women

Signs and symptoms of progesterone sensitivity include:

- Premenstrual symptoms, beginning up to three days before or during menses, including:
  - Excessive edema
  - Bloating
  - Headache
  - Depression
- Pregnancy, symptoms such as:
  - Excessive appetite
  - Excessive weight gain
  - Excessive tiredness
  - Hypertension
  - Varicose veins

Low progestational activity OCs should be chosen initially for these patients. Monophasic OCs may be helpful in lessening mood swings that may be caused by the alternating progestin doses in multiphasic OCs.

Estrogen-Deficient Women

Symptoms of estrogen insufficiency include:

- Scant menses
- Small uterus
- Small breasts
- Midcycle spotting

Women with these symptoms or findings should not be given OCs with high estrogen contents initially, as has been occasionally suggested. A lack of estrogenic effects may result from the physiological down-regulation of estrogen production; attempts to override this with excessive estrogen doses may result in undesirable side effects.

Progesterone-Deficient Women

Women with progesterone deficiency have symptoms similar to those of women with anovulatory cycles and corpus luteum insufficiency. These symptoms include:

- Prolonged menses
- Heavy menses
- Severe cramping
- Premenstrual spotting or BTB
- Premenstrual symptoms, beginning seven to 12 days before menses

Similar symptoms may occur due to endometriosis and adenomyosis. These women may require OCs with increased progestational activities.

Androgen-Sensitive Women

Women with excessive androgen effects may have:
- Very oily skin
- Acne
- Male pattern hair growth on:
  - Face
  - Abdomen below the navel
  - Midline of chest

Causes of excessive androgen effects, other than neoplasia and adrenal causes, require different treatment regimens:

- For women with high androgen and normal or high estrogen levels (polycystic or Stein-Leventhal ovaries) - High progestin/low androgen OCs for suppression
- For women with normal androgen levels and low estrogen levels who often have low levels of SSBG and, as a consequence, increased serum levels of free androgen - Balanced or estrogen-dominant OCs

#22 Implanted Contraceptives

IMPLANTS

Levonorgestrel (LNG)/Norplant®

Status

Norplant® (levonorgestrel [LNG]) is the only progestin implant approved for use in the U.S.

Contraceptive implants, made of flexible nonbiodegradable tubes filled with hormones and placed under the skin, were first developed in the 1960s. At least 10 compounds have been tested in implants. Currently, two Silastic® and one biodegradeable implants are under investigation.

Norplant® is intended to prevent pregnancy and does not protect against HIV infection, AIDS and other sexually transmitted diseases.

-FDA Package Insert Labeling

Management and Dose

Norplant® implants contain 36 mg per Silastic® capsule. Six LNG capsules, each measuring 2.4 by 34 mm, are implanted, with a 10-gauge trocar, subdermally in a fan-like pattern through a 3 to 5 mm incision in the medial aspect of the upper, volar side of the forearm.

The dose of LNG provided by the Norplant® system is initially about 85 mcg per day followed by a decline to about 50 mcg per day by nine months, about 35 mcg per day by 18 months, and a further decline thereafter to about 30 mcg per day. At three months, mean levels decline to values around 400 pg/ml, normalize to a 60 kg body weight at 327 pg/ml at 12 months, and further decline by 1.4 pg/ml per month to reach 258 pg/ml at 60 months.

Insertions should be made during the first seven days after onset of menstruation. Insertions can also be made immediately postpartum in nonnursing women and postabortion. Implants are not recommended for breastfeeding women.

Removal

Removal, performed under local anesthesia, is through a small incision. Removal is difficult if capsules are inserted too deeply. Nonpalpable capsules may be located by ultrasound.

Complications during removal were reported in 4.5 percent of 3,416 users. Most of these were related to broken or deeply imbedded implants (Ref 94).

Capsules should be removed after five years, since effectiveness decreases after that time. However, no harmful effects occur if capsules are not removed. Spontaneous expulsion occurs in the presence of infection and when insertions are too close to the incision.

A study of acceptability if U.S. users found that, although 40 percent were anxious about insertion and removal, 87 percent experienced no pain and only slight discomfort on insertion and 75 percent experienced little or no pain on removal (Ref 76). In the same study, 80 percent were satisfied with the method and 95 percent said they might use the method again.

22

Contraindications

Clinicians should take general contraindications for OCs into consideration when prescribing implants.

1. Active thrombophlebitis or thromboembolic disorders.
2. Undiagnosed abnormal genital bleeding.
3. Known or suspected pregnancy.
4. Acute liver disease; benign or malignant liver tumors.
5. Known or suspected carcinoma of the breast.
-FDA Package Insert Labeling

Clinical Information

An important reason for considering use of implants is their high continuation rate. In a study of 112 U.S. adolescents ages 18 and younger, half of whom used implants and half of whom used OCs, the continuation rate after one year was 91 percent for implant patients and 34 percent for OC users (Ref 27). As a result, 25 percent of OC users and no implant users became pregnant during that year.

Norplant® has a cumulative pregnancy rate of 3.9 per 100 women after five years, an average of 0.8 percent failures per year. The rate of release of LNG depends in part on body fat and blood supply in the area of implantation. Plasma levels of LNG are inversely related to body weight. In women who weigh 145 lbs. (70 kg) or more, pregnancy rates in the third year of use were 5.1 per 100 women and 8.5 after five years (Ref FDA Package Insert). A study in China found a similar relationship to weight, but cumulative five-year pregnancy rates were only half as high (Ref 408). In some women, dense fibrous tissue forms around the capsule.

Annual and Five-Year Cumulative Pregnancy Rates Per 100 Users by Weight Class						
	YEAR					
WEIGHT CLASS	1	2	3	4	5	Total
< 50 kg (< 110 lbs)	0.2	0	0	0	0	0.2
50-59 kg (110-130 lbs)	0.2	0.5	0.4	2.0	0.4	3.4
60-69 kg (131-153 lbs)	0.4	0.5	1.6	1.7	0.8	5.0
>70 kg (>154 lbs)	0	1.1	5.1	2.5	0	8.5
All	0.2	0.5	1.2	1.6	0.4	3.9

-FDA Package Insert Labeling

Ectopic Pregnancy

Ectopic pregnancy occurs in 1.3 per 1,000 women years, 3.0 percent of reported pregnancies. Ovulation occurs in approximately 10 percent of cycles during the first year of use and 30 to 75 percent of cycles during succeeding years.

Ectopic Pregnancies

. . . The risk of ectopic pregnancy may increase with the duration of NORPLANT SYSTEM® use and possibly with increased weight of the user. Physicians should be alert to the possibility of an ectopic pregnancy among women using the NORPLANT SYSTEM® who become pregnant or complain of lower abdominal pain. Any patient who presents with lower abdominal pain must be evaluated to rule out ectopic pregnancy. . . .

-FDA Package Insert Labeling

Bleeding Irregularities

Implants, like other progestin-only contraceptives, disrupt the menstrual cycle. The most common patient complaint is irregular bleeding, which accounts for seven to 10 percent of discontinuance during the first year of use.

One study reported disruption of the menstrual cycle in 60 to 80 percent of users in the first year (Ref 384). In a report of personal experience with 749 implant insertions, one physician reported that 23 percent of patients requested early removal. Of these, 34.3 percent of requests were because of heavy or excessive bleeding and 26.7 percent were due to a desire to become pregnant (Ref 449).

Most women can expect some variation in menstrual bleeding patterns. Irregular menstrual bleeding, intermenstrual spotting, prolonged episodes of bleeding and spotting, and amenorrhea occur in some women. Irregular bleeding patterns associated with the NORPLANT SYSTEM® could mask symptoms of cervical or endometrial cancer. Overall, these irregularities diminish with continuing use. . . .

-FDA Package Insert Labeling

Annual and Five-Year Cumulative Rates Per 100 Users						
	YEAR					
	1	**2**	**3**	**4**	**5**	**Total**
Pregnancy	0.2	0.5	1.2	1.6	0.4	3.9
Bleeding Irregularities	9.1	7.9	4.9	3.3	2.9	25.1
Medical (excluding bleeding irreg.)	6.0	5.6	4.1	4.0	5.1	22.4
Personal	4.6	7.7	11.7	10.7	11.7	38.7
Continuation	81.0	77.4	79.2	76.7	77.6	29.5

-FDA Package Insert Labeling

Bleeding irregularities decrease over time. In another study, 36 percent of women experienced bleeding for more than 31 days in the first three months. During the ninth to twelfth months, only 12 percent experienced this amount of bleeding. Higher daily release rates of LNG decrease irregular bleeding and increase amenorrhea. Despite the bleeding, total average menstrual blood loss is less than before treatment, and Hg/HCT levels rise during use.

Amenorrhea

Amenorrhea lasting more than 60 days occurs in 32 percent of cases during the first three months and in 24 percent during the ninth to twelfth months.

Delayed Follicular Atresia

In seven NDA clinical trials, temporary enlargement of the fallopian tubes and ovaries occurred in 0.8 to 4.6 percent and abdominal pains occurred in 1.7 to 8.7 percent of Norplant® users during the first year of use.

Serious Side Effects

From the introduction of implants in the U.S. in February 1991 to December 1993, the FDA received 5,800 reports of adverse events in implant users, of which 100 were serious (Ref 503). The serious events included:

- 24 hospitalizations for infection at the insertion site
- 14 reports of patients disabled because of difficult implant removal
- 14 cases of stroke
- 6 cases of thrombotic thrombocytopenia or thrombocytopenia purpura
- 39 cases of pseudotumor cerebri, of which 11 required hospitalization

Other Side Effects

In six of seven clinical trials, acne occurred in 0.6 to eight percent of Norplant® users. A higher incidence of acne occurred in one earlier trial.

Headache was doubled and nervousness was tripled in NDA trials of Norplant®, for which a control group of IUD users was included.

Fewer than one percent of patients report infections at the implantation site.

Laboratory Changes

A decrease in total cholesterol levels has been reported in all lipoprotein studies and reached statistical significance in several. Both increases and decreases in high-density lipoprotein- (HDL) cholesterol levels have been reported in clinical trials. No statically significant increases have been reported in the ratio of total cholesterol to HDL-cholesterol. Low-density lipoprotein- (LDL) cholesterol levels decreased during Norplant® use; triglyceride levels also decreased from pretreatment values.

Blood glucose levels have been shown to be elevated but within normal range. Coagulation studies show a small increase in factor VII and decrease in antithrombin III.

Other Clinical Information

Patients who develop active thrombophlebitis or thromboembolic disease should have the NORPLANT SYSTEM® capsules removed. Removal should also be considered in women who will be subjected to prolonged immobilization due to surgery or other illnesses.

-FDA Package Insert Labeling

Reference: 426

The contraceptive effect of Norplant® is reversed by removal of the implants. Time to conception is not affected by duration of use; 77 percent of users become pregnant within the first year after removal.

Most women feel little discomfort during insertion, but 30 percent have found removal painful. Minor irritation during use is reported by 10 to 12 percent. Implants are noticeable in 40 percent of women, but only seven percent consider this undesirable.

OTHER INVESTIGATIONAL IMPLANTS

Norplant-2®

Norplant-2® is currently in clinical trials. Only two rods are implanted, each measuring 2.4 by 44 mm and containing 70 mg of homogeneously dispersed LNG and covered by a layer of Silastic®.

Implanon®

Implanon® is a single ethylene vinyl acetate rod containing 3-keto-desogestrel.

Capronor®

Capronor®, a biodegradable capsule containing LNG in polycaprolactone, releases LNG 10 times faster than Silastic®, thereby requiring less surface area. Caprolactone breaks down to hydroxycapronic acid and finally to CO_2 and H_2O.

References: 25, 27, 76, 90, 94, 307, 384, 408, 426, 449, 459, 503

NOTES

#23 Injected Contraceptives

Medroxyprogesterone Acetate (MPA)/ Depo-Provera® Contraceptive Injections

Status

Depo-Provera® (MPA) is the only contraceptive injection approved for use in the U.S. MPA intramuscular (IM) has been tested extensively in the U.S. since the late 1960s and is presently used as a contraceptive in more than 90 countries.

Depo-Provera® injection is intended to prevent pregnancy and does not protect against HIV infection, AIDS, and other sexually transmitted diseases.

-FDA Package Insert Labeling

Pharmacology

MPA consists of a substituted C-21 molecule that is without androgenic or estrogenic effects. The androgenic side effects occasionally reported may be the result of decreased sex steroid binding globulin (SSBG).

MPA is a crystalline suspension that is insoluble in water and lipids. After injection, crystalline deposits form in tissue and are reabsorbed slowly. Peak levels reach 1 to 7 mg/ml three weeks after 150 mg injection. MPA may be undetectable after four months but has been measured in serum as late as eight months after injection.

Clinical Information

MPA intramuscularly (IM) is a highly effective method of contraception; its failure rate is 0.25 to 0.3 percent.

Side effects related to the progestational effect of MPA are common. The most frequent are related to the menstrual cycle, including:

- Spotting and/or breakthrough bleeding (BTB)
- Amenorrhea
- Post-use amenorrhea and/or delay in conception

Bleeding is likely to be increased at the time of surgery if a hysterectomy is performed within six weeks following postpartum in patients on Depo-Provera®.

> Most women using Depo-Provera® contraceptive injection experience disruption of menstrual bleeding patterns. Altered menstrual bleeding patterns include irregular or unpredictable bleeding or spotting, or rarely, heavy or continuous bleeding. If abnormal bleeding persists or is severe, appropriate investigation should be instituted to rule out the possibility of organic pathology, and appropriate treatment should be instituted when necessary.
>
> -FDA Package Insert Labeling

Up to 50 percent of women experience spotting or BTB during their early cycles of use. Amenorrhea frequently develops with prolonged use due to endometrial atrophy.

23

> As women continue using Depo-Provera®, fewer experience intermenstrual bleeding and more experience amenorrhea. By month 12, amenorrhea was reported by 57 percent of women, and by month 24, amenorrhea was reported by 68 percent of women using Depo-Provera®.
>
> -FDA Package Insert Labeling

Side effects occurring significantly more often with Depo-Provera® than with other means of contraception are:
- Decrease of bone density
- Weight gain

Bone Mineral Density Changes

> Use of Depo-Provera® may be considered among the risk factors for development of osteoporosis. The rate of bone loss is greater in the early years of use and then subsequently approaches the normal rate of age related fall.
>
> -FDA Package Insert Labeling

Weight Changes

> There is a tendency for women to gain weight while on Depo-Provera® therapy. From an initial average body weight of 136 lbs., women who completed one year of therapy with Depo-Provera® gained an average of 5.4 lbs. Women who completed two years of therapy gained an average of 8.1 lbs. Women who completed four years gained an average of 13.8 lbs. Women who completed six years gained an average of 16.5 lbs. Two percent of women withdrew from a large-scale clinical trial because of excessive weight gain.
>
> -FDA Package Insert Labeling

Other side effects of Depo-Provera® treatment include:

- Thromboembolic disorders
- Ocular disorders
- Fluid retention
- CNS disorders
- Convulsions

Thromboembolic Disorders

> The physician should be alert to the earliest manifestations of thrombolic disorders (thrombophlebitis, pulmonary embolism, cerebrovascular disorders, and retinal thrombosis). Should any of these occur or be suspected, the drug should not be readministered.
>
> *-FDA Package Insert Labeling*

Ocular Disorders

> Medication should not be readministered pending examination if there is a sudden partial or complete loss of vision or if there is a sudden onset of proptosis, diplopia, or migraine. If examination reveals papilledema or retinal vascular lesions, medication should not be readministered.
>
> *-FDA Package Insert Labeling*

Fluid Retention

> Because progestational drugs may cause some degree of fluid retention, conditions that might be influenced by this condition, such as epilepsy, migraine, asthma, and cardiac or renal dysfunction, require careful observation.
>
> *-FDA Package Insert Labeling*

CNS Disorders and Convulsions

> Patients who have a history of psychic depression should be carefully observed and the drug not be readministered if the depression recurs.
>
> There have been a few reported cases of convulsions in patients who were treated with Depo-Provera® contraceptive injection. Association with drug use or pre-existing conditions is not clear.
>
> *-FDA Package Insert Labeling*

Laboratory Changes

MPA causes a 25-percent decrease in triglyceride and HDL- and total cholesterol levels and causes a mild deterioration in glucose tolerance associated with an increased insulin response. Contrary to FDA labeling information, it has no effect on liver function.

Carbohydrate Metabolism

> A decrease in glucose tolerance has been observed in some patients on Depo-Provera® treatment. The mechanism of this decrease is obscure. For this reason, diabetic patients should be carefully observed while receiving such therapy.
>
> *-FDA Package Insert Labeling*

Liver Function

> If jaundice develops consideration should be given to not readministering the drug.
>
> *-FDA Package Insert Labeling*

Drug Interactions

> Aminoglutethimide administered concomitantly with the Depo-Provera® contraceptive injection may significantly depress the serum concentrations of medroxyprogesterone acetate. Depo-Provera® users should be warned of the possibility of decreased efficacy with the use of this or any related drugs.
>
> *-FDA Package Insert Labeling*

Cancer Risk
Breast Cancer

> Long-term case-controlled surveillance of Depo-Provera® contraceptive injection users found slight or no increased overall risk of breast cancer, and no overall increased risk of ovarian, liver or cervical cancer and a prolonged, protective effect of reducing the risk of endometrial cancer in the population of users. . . .
> . . . An increased relative risk (RR) of 2.19 (95 percent C.I. [confidence interval] 1.23-3.89) of breast cancer has been associated with use of Depo-Provera® in women whose first exposure to drug was within the previous four years and who were under 35 years of age. However, the overall relative risk for ever-users of Depo-Provera® was only 1.2 (95 percent C.I. 0.96-1.52). . ..
>
> *-FDA Package Insert Labeling*

Approval of Depo-Provera® IM as a contraceptive was postponed for more than two decades because of concerns about breast cancer. However, the risk appears to be small for long-term use and is balanced by a reduced risk of endometrial cancer.

After controlling for age at first birth and current age, the RR of breast cancer in ever-users of Depo-Provera® was 1.21 (Ref 490). Use before age 25 was associated with a 1.32 RR, which increased with years of total use from 1.02 for less than one year to 2.41 for more than three years. Paradoxically, the RR after age 25 was highest (1.39 to 1.42) during the first three years of use and fell to 0.78 after three years. For all ages, the risk of a newly diagnosed breast cancer was less than 1.0 eight years after first use, regardless of continuation of use.

Cervical Cancer

> . . . A statistically insignificant increase in relative risk estimates of invasive squamous cell cervical cancer has been associated with the use of Depo-Provera® in women who were first exposed before the age of 35 years (RR 1.22 to 1.28 and 95 percent C.I. 0.93-1.70). The overall, non-significant relative rate of invasive squamous cell cervical cancer in women who never used Depo-Provera was estimated to be 1.11 (95 percent C.I. 0.96-1.29). No trends in risk with duration of use or times since initial or most recent exposure were observed.
>
> *-FDA Package Insert Labeling*

Return of Fertility

> Depo-Provera® contraceptive injection has a prolonged contraceptive effect. In a large U.S. study of women who discontinued use of Depo-Provera® to become pregnant, data are available for 61 percent of them. Based on Life Table analysis of these data, it is expected than 68 percent of women who do become pregnant may conceive within 12 months, 83 percent may conceive within 15 months, and 93 percent may conceive within 18 months from the last injection. The median time to conception for those who do conceive is 10 months following the last injection with a range of four to 31 months and is unrelated to the duration of use. No data are available for 39 percent of the patients who discontinued Depo-Provera® to become pregnant and who were lost to follow-up or changed their mind.
>
> *-FDA Package Insert Labeling*

Amenorrhea and fertility may continue for an extended time after MPA IM, but the average time to return to ovulation is five to eight months and the average time to pregnancy is 10 months.

Accidental Pregnancies

Infants from accidental pregnancies that occur one to two months after injection of Depo-Provera® contraceptive injection may be at an increased risk of low birth weight, which in turn is associated with an increased risk of neonatal death. The attributable risk is low because such pregnancies are uncommon.

A significant increase in incidence of polysyndactyly and chromosomal anomalies was observed among infants of Depo-Provera® users, the former being most pronounced in women under 30 years of age. The unrelated nature of these defects, the lack of confirmation from other studies, the distant preconceptual exposure to Depo-Provera®, and the chance effects due to multiple statistical comparisons, make a causal association unlikely.

Children exposed to medroxyprogesterone acetate *in utero* and followed to adolescence, showed no evidence of any adverse effects on their health including their physical, intellectual sexual or social development.

Several reports suggest an association between intrauterine exposure to progestational drugs in the first trimester of pregnancy and genital abnormalities in male and female fetuses. The risk of hypospadias (five to eight per 1000 male births in the general population) may be approximately doubled with exposure to these drugs. There are insufficient data to quantify the risk to exposed female fetuses, but because some of these drugs induce mild virilization of the external genitalia of the female fetus and because of the increased association of hypospadias in the male fetus, it is prudent to avoid the use of these drugs during the first trimester of pregnancy.

To ensure that Depo-Provera® is not administered inadvertently to a pregnant woman, it is important that the first injection be given only during the first five days after the onset of a normal menstrual period within five days postpartum if not breast feeding and if breast feeding, at the sixth week postpartum.

-FDA Package Insert Labeling

Ectopic Pregnancy

Health-care providers should be alert to the possibility of an ectopic pregnancy among women using Depo-Provera® contraceptive injection who become pregnant or complain of severe abdominal pain.

-FDA Package Insert Labeling

Lactation

Detectable amounts of drug have been identified in the milk of mothers receiving Depo-Provera®. In nursing mothers treated with Depo-Provera® contraceptive injection, milk composition, quality, and amount are not adversely affected. Infants exposed to medroxyprogesterone via breast milk have been studied for developmental and behavioral effects through puberty. No adverse effects have been noted.

-FDA Package Insert Labeling

One of the advantages cited for MPA IM is that milk production is increased in nursing mothers. However, prolonged breastfeeding of babies whose mothers use MPA may actually have a negative effect on weight. Persistent galactorrhea for more than six months after stopping nursing was found in 64 percent of MPA users.

Management and Dose

The use of MPA IM is indicated in conditions in which estrogen-containing OCs are contraindicated and barrier methods of contraception are inadvisable when compliance is a problem and for women older than age 35 who smoke. The possibility of an extended interval until return to fertility must be understood and accepted by the patient. The author does not recommend MPA use by nursing mothers because of its uncertain effects on breastfed infants.

The usual dose of MPA is 150 mg IM every three months.

Depo-Provera® should be administered by the fifth day of menses in nonpostpartum patients and by the fifth day postpartum in nonnursing mothers.

The addition of supplemental estrogens, in either IM or oral form, for the control of irregular menstruation and amenorrhea is not recommended.

Norethindrone Enanthate (NET)

Pharmacology

NET (Schering) is the heptanoic acid ester of norethindrone, one of the 19-nor-testosterone progestins used in OCs. NET is soluble in lipids. The rate of absorption depends on the nature of the oily vehicle in which the ester is suspended.

Status

NET has been tested extensively in World Health Organization (WHO) studies since the early 1970s. There are no current plans for release in the U.S.

There are no studies linking NET use with increased risk of cancer.

Clinical Information

Use of a 60-day injection interval results in a failure rate of 0.4 percent; longer intervals, such as 84 days, markedly increase pregnancy rates. NET, when compared to MPA, has less effect on the endometrium and results in shorter menstrual cycles (especially initially after injections) and increased BTB. With continued use, cycle lengths and rates of amenorrhea increase (up to 45 percent).

Long-term use of NET results in a 25-percent reduction in HDL-cholesterol levels, a rate similar to that of MPA. No significant changes occur in glucose tolerance, though plasma insulin is increased (as with MPA) and blood pressure occasionally increases. NET has no effect on liver function.

Because of NET's appearance in breastmilk, NET is not recommended for nursing mothers. NET levels in breastmilk may reach 2 to 3 ng per ml; daily intake by a nursing infant may reach 1.5 mg per day by 60 days after injections of 200 mg.

Management and Dose

No special treatment for BTB is necessary. Patients should be advised of its likely occurrence.

The dosage of NET is 200 mg in 1 ml castor oil per benzoate 6/4 (v/v) IM every two months. The first injection should be given during menstruation, with a subsequent injection 56 to 60 days later.

References: 25, 80, 100, 142, 147, 196, 310, 312, 371, 410, 447, 484, 490, 491, 492, 493, 494, 496

#24 Emergency Contraception

General Information
The probability of conception after a single act of intercourse has been calculated to be 15 percent if it occurs once per week and increases to 33 percent if it occurs every other day. Conception probably cannot take place later than 48 hours after ovulation and possibly not later than 24 hours, but spermatozoa may survive for four to six days in the genital tract. Many women are unaware of the danger of conception following this length of time before ovulation. Emergency contraception with OCs is effective if started within 72 hours of intercourse and with copper IUDs if used within five days.

Steroidal preparations that can be used for postcoital contraception include:

- dl-Norgestrel/ethinyl estradiol combination (NG/EE)
- Levonorgestrel/ethinyl estradiol combination (LN/EE)
- dl-Norgestrel (NG)
- Ethinyl estradiol (EE)
- Mifepristone (RU 486)
- Conjugated estrogen (CE) (oral and intravenous)

Copper-wrapped IUDs can prevent pregnancy, with a failure rate of less than one percent, when used as late as five days after ovulation (Ref 134).

Pharmacology
EE, a component of many OCs, NG, and LN are discussed in Section #3. RU 486 is a synthetic 19-norsteroid with potent antiprogestational and antiglucocorticoid properties used in some countries for medical induction of abortion during the first 63 days of gestation.

Status
Use of NG/EE, LN/EE, NG, EE, CE and RU 486 for postcoital contraception are presently awaiting approval by the FDA.

Clinical Information

To be effective, postcoital contraceptive agents must be administered as soon as possible after unprotected coital exposure. When administered within 72 hours of intercourse, recognizable pregnancy occurs only 0.6 percent or less of the time compared to an expected rate of two to 30 percent. Initiation of regimens within 24 hours of intercourse increases the chance that pregnancy will be prevented.

Marked nausea and vomiting are common with sex steroid regimens and RU 486 but least of all with LN. For this reason, it is recommended that patients be observed for up to seven hours after taking treatment. Additional tablets should be prescribed to replace those lost due to vomiting. Antinausea medications may also be given.

Irregular bleeding may follow treatment. Menses is delayed four to 63 days in half of women who take RU 486 prior to ovulation and in 16 percent who take it after ovulation mistakenly. Early bleeding may occur after all regimens including RU 486.

A 1997 study found that, while more than half of American women had heard of emergency contraception, 55 percent did not know it was available in the U.S. (Ref 295). The same study found that only five percent of women had learned about emergency contraception from their physicians and that only 10 percent of obstetrician/gynecologists had discussed emergency contraception with their patients. A 1998 survey of U.K. emergency room physicians found that less than 10 percent always prescribed emergency contraception when requested or indicated, that 39 percent never did, and that 45 percent prescribed it only if a patient could not be seen by an obstetrician/gynecologist within 72 hours (Ref 283).

Management and Dose

The usual doses are:

- NG/EE - 0.5/0.05 mg two tablets repeated 12 hours later or four tablets in a single dose

- LN/EE – 0.15/0.03 mg three of four tablets repeated in 12 hours
- NG - 0.075 mg six tablets repeated in 12 hours
- EE - 2.5 mg orally twice daily for five days
- CE - 10 mg orally three times a day for five days
- CE - 25 mg IV immediately and repeated in 24 hours
- RU 486 - 600 mg as a single dose (three 200 mg or tablets)

Although none of the postcoital methods are currently FDA-approved, there are circumstances, such as rape or failure of barrier contraception, in which these methods are needed.

Pregnancy Rates

The failure rate with high-dose oral estrogens was 0.3 percent in 9,000 cases, 10 percent of which were ectopic pregnancies. The failure rate with NG/EE was at 0.6 percent in 1,300 cases, with no ectopic pregnancies. The failure rate with IV Premarin® has been reported as 3.3 percent.

In comparative double blind studies, the pregnancy rate of four percent for NG/EE (in a regimen of four tablets in a single dose) was significantly lower than the rate of nine percent for EE (in a regimen of 5 mg tablets for five days). Nausea and vomiting occurred in 16 percent and 21 percent, respectively. In another study, pregnancy rates were equal for NG/EE and LN/EE and nausea was much less for LN.

In a double blind study, there were no pregnancies with RU 486 vs one percent with NG/EE. Nausea was higher, 60 percent with NG/EE vs 40 percent with RU 486. Delayed menses occurred in 42 percent of recipients with RU 486 vs 16 percent with NG/EE.

Patients who remain pregnant after treatment may be at increased risk of birth defects. However, the possibility of birth defects as a result of short-term postcoital drug therapy is small. RU 486 has caused sirenomelia, or the mermaid syndrome, in which the legs are fused.

References: 68, 134, 135, 181, 295, 332, 448, 506, 507

NOTES

#25 Other Hormonal and Developmental Contraceptives

Progestin-Filled Intrauterine Devices
Vaginal Rings
GnRH Agonists and Antagonists
Male Contraception

PROGESTIN-FILLED INTRAUTERINE DEVICES
Progestasert ®

Status

The Progestasert Intrauterine Progesterone Contraceptive System® (Alza) is available in both the U.S. and Canada.

Clinical Information

The contraceptive effectiveness of the Progestasert® is roughly the same as for other intrauterine devices (IUDs), about 1.2 to 1.4 pregnancies per 100 women per years (WYS) of use. The incidence of ectopic pregnancy is higher than that of OCs and other IUDs.

The contraceptive effects of progestin-filled IUDs are localized to the uterus, endometrium, and, possibly, cervical mucus. The amount of menstrual bleeding and severity of menstrual cramps are reported to be decreased with progestin-filled IUDs as compared to patients' normal patterns and to other IUDs. However, intermenstrual spotting is usually increased and continuous spotting is common; both effects are due to the localized effect of progesterone on the endometrium.

Management and Dose

The dosage of Progestasert® is 38 mg of progesterone in a silicone oil base, released at a rate of 65 mcg per day. The Progestasert® must be replaced yearly in order to maintain effectiveness. Such need for annual replacement and frequency of spotting make the Progestasert® less desirable than other IUDs for most patients, despite the reported compensatory decreases in total amounts of menstrual flow and dysmenorrhea.

Patients needing hormonal contraception without extra risks of estrogen may choose the progestin-only mini-pill, which is as effective as the Progestasert® and has similar bleeding and spotting effects, or medroxyprogesterone acetate (MPA) intramuscular injections, which offer markedly greater effectiveness and a slightly lower incidence of bleeding.

VAGINAL RINGS
LNG 20 IUD

Status
The LNG 20 IUD manufactured in Finland and used in many countries is not available in the U.S. The LNG 20 releases 20 mcg of levonorgestrel per day and is effective for seven years.

Clinical Information

25.

In a trial of more than 1,100 women in five clinics, the failure rate of the LNG 20 IUD over seven years was 1.1 percent. In another trial of 1,821 women in 14 clinics, its failure rate over three years of use was 0.3 percent. The LNG 20 appears to have a lower incidence of ectopic pregnancy than progestin-filled IUDs.

Management
Menstrual bleeding is reduced with the LNG 20 IUD, and amenorrhea may occur.

GnRH AGONISTS AND ANTAGONISTS

Clinical Information
Luteinizing hormone-releasing hormone (LHRH) agonists and antagonists are potent drugs that block ovulation. Clinical use of these agents in the U.S. is limited to treatment for prostatic cancer. In Europe, gonadotropin-releasing hormone (GnRH) analogs are used for:

- Suppression of ovarian cysts
- Regulation of ovarian response for *in vitro* fertilization
- Human gonadotropin stimulation
- Suppression of uterine fibroids
- Treatment of endometriosis

Status

Clinical trials for GnRH for treatment of endometriosis are ongoing in the U.S. Their prolonged use at doses that result in complete ovarian suppression causes osteoporosis and depressed HDL-cholesterol levels.

GnRH analogs are not effective for the induction of abortion.

The future use of these agents for contraception is doubtful at this time.

Management and Dose

Doses used for contraception are 200 to 400 mcg per day nasally in a single dose, with more potent agonists used in doses as low as 125 mcg/day. Long-acting injections may be possible.

Bleeding irregularities are common with use of these agents. Nasal irritation may occur.

MALE CONTRACEPTION

Steroids

Although trials of hormonal and nonhormonal male contraceptive pills and injections have been conducted for many years, none are close to release for clinical use.

Spermatogenesis, male body characteristics, and the male sex act depend on the presence of male hormones, principally testosterone; but attempts to suppress active testosterone or the pituitary gonadotropins in order to prevent spermatogenesis inevitably alter the male sexual response and male body characteristics.

Significant side effects can occur, including increased risks of:
- Liver cancer
- Prostate cancer
- Cardiovascular disease

Steroid drugs used for male contraception include:
- Depomedroxyprogesterone acetate (DMPA)
- Testosterone enanthate
- DMPA + testosterone cypionate
- 17-ß-hydroxyprogesterone acetate + testosterone enanthate
- 19-nor-testosterone IM
- LNG (oral) + testosterone enanthate
- Cyproterone acetate

Management and Dose
Steroid drugs are administered every two to four weeks. Azoospermia is usually noted seven to 13 weeks after commencing treatment and may persist for four to 20 weeks after the last injection.

GnRH Analogs for Males
When GnRH analogs are used alone, impotence often occurs. Because of this, testosterone derivatives are usually added.

GnRH analogs must be taken daily as injection or nasal inhalation preparations.

Nonsteroids
Gossypol, a derivative of cottonseed, is 99-percent effective for male contraception after two to three months of use. Male fertility usually returns six months after discontinuing treatment but may require two to three years. Permanent sterility remains in 10 percent of patients.

Inhibin, a natural protein found in semen, suppresses follicle-stimulating hormone (FSH) while stimulating spermatogenesis. Inhibin may inhibit sperm production without causing impotence.

Anticancer Drugs

Anticancer drugs that have been tested for male contraception include:

- Tetramine (TEM)
- Triethylenethiophosphoramide (TEPA)
- Nitrofuran
- Busulfan and other esters of sulfonic acids

References: 90, 91, 102, 122, 296, 389, 423

NOTES

UTERINE CHANGES

Carcinoma of the Reproductive Organs
  Numerous epidemiological studies have been performed on the incidence of breast, endometrial, ovarian, and cervical cancers in women using oral contraceptives. . . .
  In spite of many studies of the relationship between oral contraceptive use and breast or cervical cancer, a cause and effect relationship has not been established.

-FDA Package Insert Labeling

Endometrial Cancer

The risk of developing endometrial cancer is reduced 50 percent after one year of OC use, decreases further with increasing length of use, and continues to be reduced for at least 15 years after discontinuing OCs. Furthermore, this protection extends to adenocarcinoma, adenoacanthoma, and adenosquamous lesions (Ref 285). Protection has been reported for all monophasic OCs, including those with less than 50 mcg ethinyl estradiol (EE). Thus far, insufficient data have been collected on multiphasic OCs to determine if they also provide protection.

A 1995 meta-analysis found the risk of endometrial cancer to be 438 per 100,000 women for never-users ages 20 to 54. For women using OCs for eight years, the risk was decreased by 197 cases (Ref 368). The risk of endometrial cancer in both users and nonusers is low. A meta-analysis estimated that the risk of nonusers developing endometrial cancer through age 74 was 2.4 percent compared to 1.4 percent for women who had used OCs for 12 years (Ref 369). Another analysis estimated that the number of cases of endometrial cancer per 100,000 U.S. women would be decreased by 270 over their lifetimes if they used OCs for five years (Ref 318). Yet another analysis estimated that use of OCs for eight years or longer would result in 1,900 fewer cases of endometrial cancer in the U.S. (Ref 318). However, one researcher estimated that, for 100,000 women who used OCs continuously from ages 16 to 35, there would be only 10 fewer deaths from endometrial cancer over their lifetimes (Ref 451). These reductions must be balanced against a possible increase in breast and cervical cancers. Use of OCs for 12 years increased the probability of being free of endometrial cancer to 98.6 percent (cancer risk of 1.4 percent) (Ref 369).

Studies of endometrial carcinoma have reported an increased risk associated with prolonged administration of exogenous estrogen to postmenopausal women. In a report on the first 21 cases submitted by physicians to a registry of cases of adenocarcinoma of the endometrium in OC users younger than age 40, almost all cases in patients without predisposing factors for endometrial cancer (irregular bleeding before OC use, polycystic ovaries) occurred in those taking sequential OCs. These products are no longer marketed.

Cyclic administration of progestins alone or in combination with OCs may reduce risks of endometrial cancer in women who do not ovulate regularly.

References: 51, 195, 424, 368, 369

26.

Leiomyomata
Clinical Information

Uterine size and the size of pre-existing leiomyomata may either increase or decrease, depending on the estrogen activity of a particular OC and the sensitivity of the individual.

Cellular atypia may occur in myomas of OC users. However, a definite relationship between OC hormones and atypical myomas cannot be demonstrated. Myomas with multifocal hemorrhages (apoplectic leiomyomas) may be more common in OC users. Reported symptoms include:

- Acute or chronic pain
- Dysmenorrhea
- Hemoperitoneum
- Vaginal bleeding

Symptoms usually develop after two to four years of OC use. Pain may be sufficient to require laparotomy.

There is no evidence that OC use causes the formation of new leiomyomata. The incidence of clinically apparent leiomyomata was shown to decrease in OC users in a large prospective study.

In one study of 55 premenopausal women with leiomyomatas who used OCs containing 30 to 35 mcg EE and ethynodiol diacetate 1 mg, desogestrel 0.15 mg, norethindrone 1 mg, or norgestrel 0.3 mg for one year, no increase in size was found on repeat ultrasound (Ref 123).

Causal Factors

The myometrium is one of the most sensitive tissues to the stimulation of estrogen. Estrogen causes both a real growth of myometrial cells and edema.

The endometrium grows in response to the estrogen component. Pre-existing uterine leiomyomata may increase in size in the presence of excess estrogen and may decrease if estrogenic activity is low. Progestins, with the exception of norethynodrel, may cause a decrease in leiomyoma size.

The progestin component causes:
- Glycogen deposition in the cells of endometrial glands
- A coiling of arterioles
- Other changes that mature the endometrium and facilitate shedding of all but the basal layer at the time of menstruation

Management

Appropriate diagnostic measures should be taken to rule out malignancy, if undiagnosed vaginal bleeding before beginning or during OC use is:
- Persistent
- Recurrent
- Abnormal

If leiomyoma growth is noted, patients should be switched to OCs with lower estrogenic activities. If regression in size does not occur, the possibility of uterine or ovarian neoplasia or pregnancy must be considered. GnRH agonists produce temporary reductions in leiomyoma size because they reduce ovarian estrogen production to menopausal levels. GnRH agonists should not be administered simultaneously with OCs since each will counteract the effect of the other.

References: 83, 84, 108, 123, 205, 248, 282, 356, 381, 388, 477, 510

OVARIAN CHANGES

Ovarian Cysts
In general, the incidence of benign ovarian cysts is reduced in OC users. However, there are several reports of the development of follicular and corpus luteum cysts, some very large, in patients using triphasic and low-dose monophasic OCs (Ref 45, 56, 505). In one report, the OCs used were:

- Triphasil® for 12 patients
- Ortho-Novum 7/7/7® for three patients
- Ortho-Novum 10/11® for two patients
- Not indicated for two patients

Several patients received surgery to remove these cysts. However, in all cases in which patients switched to high-progesterone potency monophasic OCs, the cysts resolved.

In a randomized, controlled study, the risk of developing a functional ovarian cyst (larger than 3.0 mm) during OC use was equal for low-dose monophasic and triphasic OCs and twice as large as for higher-dose monophasic OCs (odds ratio [OR] = 0.5) (Ref 152).

Ovarian Cancer
The incidence of ovarian cancer is reduced in OC users. This protective effect increases with years of use from 14 percent after one year to 50 percent after five years (Ref 118). Protection is greatest in women younger than age 25. The risk reduction occurs with all monophasic OCs and extends to serous, endometrial,

and clear cell tumors. It is uncertain if mucinous tumors are prevented (Ref 51).

Women using OCs have only 60 percent of the risk of developing ovarian cancer compared to nonusers of the same age, and this reduced risk appears to persist for as long as 10 years after discontinuing OC use. The reduction of risk increases as the duration of OC use increases and is 60 percent for women who use OCs for more than five years.

Ovarian cancer occurs in about four percent of U.S. women. The natural incidence is increased in women of low parity and, possibly, with familial predispositions to ovarian cancer.

A 1995 meta-analysis estimated the risk of developing ovarian cancer in never-users ages 20 and 54 to be 369 per 100,000 women. For women using OCs for eight years, the estimated risk was decreased by 193 cases (Ref 368). Another analysis estimated that the number of cases of ovarian cancer per 100,000 U.S. women would be decreased by 215 cases over their lifetimes if they used OCs for five years (Ref 62). Yet another analysis estimated that use of OCs for eight years or longer would result in 1,000 fewer cases of ovarian cancer in the U.S. (Ref 318). However, one researcher estimated that, for 100,000 women who used OCs continuously from ages 16 to 35, there would be only 140 fewer deaths from ovarian cancer over their lifetimes (Ref 451). These reductions must be balanced against a possible increase in breast and cervical cancers.

References: 45, 51, 56, 62, 118, 168, 318, 348, 356, 368, 390, 397, 401, 451, 461, 473, 478, 505

NOTES

#27 Breast Disorders

Breast Symptoms
Fibrocystic Breast Disease
Breast Cancer

Carcinoma of the Breast
    . . . The evidence in the literature suggests that use of oral contraceptives is not associated with an increase in the risk of developing breast cancer, regardless of the age and parity of first use or with most of the marketed brands and doses. The Cancer and Steroid Hormone study also showed no latent effect on the risk of breast cancer for at least a decade following long-term use. A few studies have shown a slightly increased relative risk of developing breast cancer, although the methodology of these studies, which included differences in examination of users and non-users and differences in age at start of use, has been questioned. Some studies have reported an increased relative risk of developing breast cancer, particularly at a younger age. This increased relative risk appears to be related to duration of use.

-FDA Package Insert Labeling

BREAST SYMPTOMS

Clinical Information
Breast symptoms include the following:
- Breast pain (mastalgia)
- Breast tenderness
- Swelling

Swelling and breast tenderness are common premenstrual symptoms and occur frequently in women using high estrogen- and high progestin-dose OCs. The incidence of breast symptoms seems to be decreased in women using low-dose formulations.

Causal Factors
Breast symptoms may be due to:
- Edema
- Growth of breast tissue
- Infection
- Vascular congestion

Management

When breast tenderness and swelling occur but are not unilateral or are accompanied by palpable masses, switching patients to OCs with lower estrogen potencies or lower progestin contents is indicated. These patients should be instructed to reduce their caffeine and sodium intakes. A diuretic may also provide temporary relief of symptoms.

If symptoms persist, further evaluation is required.

References: 83, 87, 88, 108, 198

FIBROCYSTIC BREAST DISEASE

Clinical Information

Fibrocystic breast disease (FCBD) may include any of the following diagnoses:
- Breast nodules
- Fibrocystic disease
- Fibroadenomas
- Fibroadenosis

The original observation of the Royal College of General Practitioners (RCGP) study that the total incidence of benign nodules of the breast requiring breast biopsies (fibroadenosis and fibrocystic disease) is reduced by 50 percent in patients after the second year of OC use has been confirmed by others. Ory and others found a 30-percent reduction in FCBD after one to two years of OC use and a 65-percent reduction after two years.

However, other studies have not found OCs to be protective against the development of fibrocystic breast disease that requires breast biopsy. One study found an increased occurrence of benign breast disease in postmenopausal women who were former OC users.

Causal Factors

Estrogen stimulates breast tissue growth directly by acting on the breast tissue and indirectly by stimulation of prolactin production. Progestins antagonize these

27.

effects of the estrogen component. This antagonism is greatest in OCs with high progestational and/or androgenic activities.

Occasionally, OC users experience an increase in breast size and in benign breast nodules (fibroadenomas and fibrocystic disease) due to individual estrogen sensitivity.

Management

Women should be carefully monitored if they elect to use OCs and have strong family histories of:

- Breast nodules
- Fibrocystic disease
- Breast cancer

Women who experience bilateral breast pain or masses without edema while taking OCs should be switched to OCs with lesser amounts of both estrogen and progestin and be examined for malignancy.

If pain is due to edema, patients should be switched to OCs with progestins that have less androgenic activities or lower estrogen doses. If pain continues or if masses fail to decrease in size within one month, OCs should be discontinued until malignancy can be ruled out by appropriate tests.

Possible breast neoplasia should be considered in women who develop unilateral breast pain or masses. These patients should be advised to discontinue OCs and use other contraceptive methods until a diagnosis is established.

References: 29, 35, 87, 88, 107, 108, 109, 119, 179, 243, 308, 356, 358, 398, 456

BREAST CANCER

Clinical Information

The risk of developing breast cancer for women up to age 80 is estimated at one in eight.

Collaborative Group Studies

The Collaborative Group on Hormonal Factors in Breast Cancer may have published the definitive study on breast cancer and OC use in June 1996 (Ref 65). This meta-analysis includes 53,297 women with breast cancer and 100,239 controls from 54 studies conducted in 25 countries. The key findings were that:

- There is a small increase in the relative risk (RR) of having breast cancer diagnosed while combined OCs are taken and up to 10 years following discontinuance
- There is no increased excess risk of diagnosis 10 years or more after OCs are discontinued
- Cancers diagnosed in women who used combined OCs were less advanced clinically than those diagnosed in women who had never used OCs
- Breast cancers diagnosed in ever users were less clinically advanced than those diagnosed in never users for up to 20 years after discontinuing OCs

There was no significant variation in RR associated with specific types of estrogen or progestin. When grouped according to hormone dose, there was a decreased risk of diagnosed breast cancer with increasing estrogen dose among women who had discontinued use 10 years before. The author concludes that these results are incompatible with a genotoxic effect but are perhaps compatible with the concept that OCs may promote the growth of cancers already initiated. They also suggest that the decreased risk, seen in certain groups 10 years after OCs were discontinued, may be analogous to the protective effect of childbearing on breast cancer risk.

Previous Studies

Previous studies have shown either a slight increase or a possible protective effect against breast cancer for OC users, after adjusting for other risk factors. One review of 22 epidemiological studies found no increased risk in OC users. Another also found no adverse effect on the progression of breast cancer among women taking

OCs at the time of diagnosis. Dr. Clifford Kay, after further analysis of the RCGP study, concluded that the study's results were incompatible with the opinion that OCs initiated breast cancer but were compatible with accelerated clinical presentation of breast cancer (Ref 479).

A population-based, case control study in the U.S. found a modest increase in breast cancer in women who began OC use within five years of menarche (odds ratio [OR] = 1.3) or used OCs for more than 10 years (OR = 1.7) (Ref 479). The author speculates that long-term OC use among young women who start use near menarche may be associated with a small excess of breast cancer risk, possibly due to genetic damage in breast epithelial cells at a time of rapid breast cell proliferation.

A former U.K. national case control study group reported an increased risk of breast cancer associated with OC use if the cancer was diagnosed before age 36. In these women, the RR was 1.43 for women who used OCs for more than four years (49 to 96 months) and was 1.74 for women who used OCs for more than eight years (96 months).

History of Benign Breast Disease

A history of benign breast disease was found to be associated with a higher incidence of breast cancer in two studies, but the opposite effect was found in other studies.

Estrogen and Progestin Dose

One study in 1983 purported to link breast cancer in young women to OCs with high progestin doses and use of OCs before age 25. These findings could not be confirmed in other studies, and the relationship of breast cancer to progestin content was not seen in the original study when more accurate means of estimating progestin doses were used.

A large U.S. case control study found no relationship of breast cancer to the dose of estrogen or progestin or to length of use. A 1994 case control study from the

Netherlands found the RR of breast cancer was greater for low-dose (less than 50 mcg) estrogen OCs than for those with 50 mcg or more of estrogen, particularly when used for more than eight years (Ref 344). In the same study, no relationship was found with progestin type or dose when adjusted for length of use. A 1992 epidemiological review also found no relationship to progestin type or dose in OC or hormone replacement therapy users (Ref 399). A protective and therapeutic effect of progesterone and progestins in breast cancer has been suggested (Ref 128).

Neither the relationship to high-progestin dose nor the use of OCs before birth of a first child before age 25 could be confirmed by a large U.S. study. The same study found no increased risk even in women who used OCs for six years before age 25.

Other Risk Factors

The effect of family history of breast cancer was not synergistic according to two studies. No positive relationship between breast cancer and **caffeine** use has been found, although a relationship to benign breast disease is known. Another study reported that women who used OCs before their **first term** birth had an increased risk of developing breast cancer before age 45. Among subgroups of women who used OCs for more than four years and who developed breast cancer before age 36, the risk was increased for **alcohol** users vs nonusers. A family history of breast cancer was also associated with increased risk (3.5 vs 1.43), while the risk was decreased with increasing **body weight** after adjustments for age at menarche, nulliparity, age at first term pregnancy, and breastfeeding. Another study, not as well controlled for additional risk factors, found the opposite effect, i.e., a decreased risk of breast cancer with **alcohol** use.

Incidence

A 1995 meta-analysis estimated the risk of developing breast cancer from ages 20 to 54 in never-users to be 2,782 per 100,000 women per years (WYS).

For women using OCs for eight years, the estimated number of additional cases of breast cancer was 151 per 100,000 WYS (Ref 368). Another analysis estimated that the number of cases of breast cancer per 100,000 U.S. women would be increased by 134 cases over their lifetimes if they used OCs for five years (Ref 62). Yet another analysis estimated that use of OCs for eight years or longer would result in 600 additional cases of breast cancer in the U.S. (Ref 318). However, one researcher estimated that, for 100,000 women who used OCs continuously from ages 16 to 35, there would be an additional 31 to 416 deaths from breast cancer over their lifetimes (Ref 451). These potential increases must be balanced against a 50-percent decrease in endometrial and cervical cancers.

Causal Factors

The cause of breast cancer is unknown, as is believed to be true for most other cancers. Inciting agents may take 20 years to be clinically expressed. Long-term continuous administration of either natural or synthetic estrogen in certain animal species increases the frequency of carcinoma of:

- Breast
- Cervix
- Vagina
- Liver

Women are known to be at increased risk of developing breast cancer if they:

- Have family histories of breast cancer in first-order relatives
- Have histories of biopsies for benign breast disease
- Are nulliparous or had first term pregnancies at ages 25 or older
- Achieved menarche before age 12
- Were never breastfed

Women with none of these factors are considered to be at low risk. Those who have one factor are at medium risk. Those with two or more factors are at high risk.

Synthetic progestins used in OCs have not, though other synthetic progestins used in injections have, been noted to increase the incidence of benign and malignant mammary nodules in dogs.

Women using combination OCs exhibited an increased frequency of sister-chromatid exchange in one study.

Pre-existing neoplasms may increase in size and become more easily noticed in some women after they start OCs. Conversely, breasts may become smaller in patients taking low estrogen OCs, while nonhormone-sensitive neoplasms remain unchanged in size.

The question of a relationship between OC use and breast cancer is not likely to be resolved in the near future, due to the prolonged time required for cancer to develop. To date, it is not known which receptors may be responsible for hormone effects on breast cancer and whether estrogens, progestins, or their metabolites act on them.

Management

Women with unilateral breast pain or masses should discontinue OCs and use different contraception methods until a diagnosis of possible breast neoplasm is either confirmed or refuted. A breast mass that appears for the first time while OCs are being taken should be considered malignant until proven otherwise.

It is now recommended that all women have mammograms upon reaching age 40 and at one- to two-year intervals thereafter. Patients with symptoms of pain and change in breast size should be examined for malignancy and a mammogram should be performed. For all patients, it is prudent for clinicians to perform breast examinations at least annually.

Mammography is relatively insensitive in younger women. Only 45 percent of histologically confirmed breast cancers in women younger than age 36 presenting with discrete masses were diagnosed by mammography compared to 78 percent diagnosed by fine needle aspiration (Ref 504). In the same study, 16 percent of patients with cancer had negative results on clinical examination, mammography, and fine needle aspiration. When all other investigations yield negative results, excision biopsy is mandatory in women with discrete breast masses.

Women at medium and high risks who are of low body weight and have strong family histories of breast cancer should be carefully monitored by breast examinations and mammograms, regardless of OC use.

Women younger than age 36 who use OCs for more than four years, are of low body weight, and consume alcohol may be at additional risk for breast cancer.

Several ongoing studies suggest that OCs may be used safely by patients who have breast cancer (Ref 170).

The issue of whether an association between OC use and breast cancer exists may have been answered. An increased incidence of breast cancer may exist; but if it does, the incidence is small in relation to the numerous benefits of OC use, including a reduction of ovarian and endometrial cancers. Furthermore, women diagnosed as having breast cancer while taking OCs may take some comfort in the fact that their tumors are less likely to have spread and that earlier diagnosis may result in higher cure rates than for never-users. Women who have not borne children before age 30 may be encouraged by the finding that OC use before age 30 may provide the same protective effect as having had a child.

References: 10, 35, 36, 49, 50, 52, 55, 60, 62, 65, 103, 107, 128, 129, 141, 144, 170, 172, 179, 184, 202, 207, 212, 244, 257, 265, 266, 276, 277, 281, 318, 344, 345, 351, 368, 370, 397, 398, 399, 437, 439, 451, 452, 455, 456, 462, 468, 504

NOTES

#28 Post-Pill Amenorrhea/Galactorrhea

> Some women may encounter post-pill amenorrhea or oligomenorrhea, especially when such a condition was pre-existent.
>
> *-FDA Package Insert Labeling*

Amenorrhea is the absence of menses. Galactorrhea is the abnormal discharge of milk or fluid from the breast and may only be detectable by squeezing the nipple.

Clinical Information

When high-estrogen content OCs were first introduced in the early 1960s, post-pill amenorrhea (PPA) and post-pill amenorrhea with galactorrhea (PPAG) were frequent sequelae of OC use. Amenorrhea was usually self-limiting and could last for up to 12 months, but menses usually returned within three months. As estrogen doses were lowered, PPA and PPAG occurred less frequently and are now rarely seen.

Causal Factors

PPA and PPAG after discontinuing OC use may be the result of:

- Hyperplasia of lactotrope cells/increased prolactin (15.7 percent)
- Use of psychotropic drugs
- Increased thyroid-stimulating hormone (TSH) due to hypothyroidism
- A prolactin or growth hormone-secreting pituitary adenoma (6.7 percent)
- Hypothalamic deficiency (51.2 percent)

Increased prolactin levels can occur when OCs containing as little as 35 mcg ethinyl estradiol (EE) are used but are usually associated with OCs containing 50 mcg or higher EE.

Estrogen present in OCs stimulates prolactin secretion by a direct action on pituitary lactotroph cells.

Prolactin prevents ovulation and menstruation by inhibiting gonadotropin-releasing hormone (GnRH) production by the hypothalamus and by blocking the ovarian response to luteinizing hormone (LH).

Use of psychotropic drugs may lead to increased prolactin production by blocking the production or action of dopamine, a natural prolactin inhibitor in the central nervous system (CNS). These drugs include:

- Reserpine
- Phenothiazines
- Tricyclic antidepressants (see Ref 88 for complete list)

Primary hypothyroidism results in high levels of TSH, which directly stimulates prolactin production by the lactotrope cells. Mild hypothyroidism occurs fairly frequently in women of reproductive age. Symptoms of hypothyroidism (e.g., weight gain or tiredness) may erroneously be attributed to OC use or may be masked by OCs (in cases of irregular menses or amenorrhea).

Pituitary adenoma may be present in up to 24 percent of PPAG patients, whereas its incidence in patients with spontaneously-occurring amenorrhea with galactorrhea is 55 percent. There is no evidence that OC users are more likely to develop pituitary adenomas than nonusers.

Intramuscular progestins used for contraception **28.** increase the amount of milk production and may induce amenorrhea for up to six months. The length of amenorrhea is dose-dependent. Breakthrough bleeding may occur instead of amenorrhea.

Failure of menses to return after discontinuing OC use may be due to:

- Pregnancy
- Polycystic ovaries (PCO) (16.6 percent)
- Ovarian failure/menopause
- Physiological factors, e.g., starvation, excessive exercise (12.8 percent)
- Obesity (weight gain greater than 30 lbs.)
- Psychological factors (e.g., anorexia)

- Nonprolactin or growth hormone-producing pituitary adenoma
- Premature menopause (3.8 percent)
- Any factors causing PPAG (5.1 percent)

Women (except those with PCO) who had irregular menses before taking OCs are more likely to have amenorrhea after discontinuing OC use. PCO patients may have one or two regular ovulatory cycles and may become pregnant immediately after discontinuing OCs before resuming their pre-OC patterns of menses every three to six months.

Amenorrhea that occurs during OC use is frequently due to inadequate hormone content; however, pregnancy may also be the cause (see Section #9).

Management

If PPAG is present, evaluation should proceed at once.

If PPA is the only symptom, it is acceptable to wait for spontaneous return of menses after elimination of possible causes, such as:

- Pregnancy
- Pituitary disorders
- Thyroid disease
- Psychotropic drug use

Patients should use barrier methods if they desire contraception while waiting for spontaneous resumption of menses.

Women with pre-existing amenorrhea prior to OC use should be advised of the possibility that amenorrhea may return after they discontinue OC use and should be encouraged to use other contraceptive methods if they discontinue OCs. PPA, possibly prolonged, may also occur in women without previous irregularities.

Evaluation of PPAG and PPA should be started three months after OCs are discontinued if PPA is the only symptom but may be delayed further if oligomenorrhea was present before OC use.

Tests should include:

- Quantitative human chorionic gonadotropin (hCG)
- Serum follicle stimulating hormone (FSH) and E_2 to rule out menopause
- Serum prolactin
- TSH or free T_4

Serum prolactin levels may be interpreted as follows:

- 35 ng/ml - Prolactin-secreting tumor not present
- 36 to 200 ng/ml – Probable lactotrophe hyperplasia but may indicate prolactin-secreting tumor; prolactin levels should be repeated in six months:
  - If repeat prolactin is greater than 50 ng/ml, a pituitary serial tomogram, CAT scan, or MRI is indicated; if these are negative, prolactin levels should be repeated every six to 12 months
  - Tomograms and CAT scans should be repeated only if prolactin levels rise (cataracts may result from repeated use)
- Greater than 200 ng/ml – Probable pituitary adenoma. Plain sella turcica x-rays should be performed first. If inconclusive, serial tomogram, CAT scan, or MRI should be performed to determine if a suprasellar turcica tumor is present. If results are still negative, prolactin levels should be repeated six to 12 months later

Treatment

Bromocryptine (Parlodel®, Sandoz) has been the treatment of choice for many years for patients with prolactin-secreting tumors and those with pituitary hyperplasia and amenorrhea who desire pregnancy. Recently, other drugs that can be taken orally daily, e.g., peroglide mesylate (Permax®) or twice weekly cabergolise (Dostinex®) have been introduced.

The dose of bromocriptine is 1.25 mg (one-half tablet) every eight hours or 2.5 mg every 12 hours daily until menses occurs or until ovulation is detected by basal body temperature (BBT).

Menses resumes in an average of five weeks after beginning therapy but may be delayed for several months if prolactin levels are high. Patients who fail to ovulate with prolactine-suppressing drugs alone may respond when clomiphene citrate 50 to 100 mg daily for five days is added.

After menses is re-established, prolactin-suppressing drugs may only be needed for the first two weeks of each cycle, thereby avoiding medication after conception has occurred.

Common side effects of bromocriptine therapy include nausea and dizziness. Less common side effects include constipation and sinus headaches. Side effects are greatly reduced when one-half tablet is taken every eight hours instead of one tablet every 12 hours.

Pregnancy

During pregnancy, the pituitary expands and nonsymptomatic adenomas may become symptomatic and cause headaches or pressure on the optic nerve and partial loss of vision. A neurosurgeon should be consulted before a decision is made regarding management of pituitary adenoma. Currently, bromocriptine use to decrease the size of prolactin-secreting pituitary adenoma is preferred over surgical removal of the adenoma.

Because pregnancy may occur spontaneously before the resumption of menses, a pregnancy test should be repeated before any additional diagnostic tests or treatments that could have adverse effects on the conceptus are instituted.

References: 84, 85, 88, 109, 110, 200, 326

NOTES

#29 Nutritional and Weight Changes

Nutritional Changes
Weight Increase or Decrease
Dietary and Exercise Amenorrhea
Changes in Laboratory Values

NUTRITIONAL CHANGES

Clinical Information

OCs may decrease serum levels of:

- Folacin (folic acid)*
- Pyridoxine (vitamin B_6)
- Riboflavin (vitamin B_2)
- Cobalamin (vitamin B_{12})
- Thiamine (vitamin B_1)
- Ascorbic acid (vitamin C)
- Calcitriol (vitamin D)
- Tocopherol (Vitamin E)
- Zinc
- Magnesium

*One study found increased levels.

Regardless of lowered vitamin and mineral levels, routine use of multivitamin supplements is usually unnecessary for OC users. Low levels of vitamin B_6, however, can cause depression and impaired glucose tolerance, a loss that can be adequately corrected by daily supplementation of 10 mg vitamin B_6.

One study measured folic acid, retinol (vitamin A), thiamine (vitamin B_1), riboflavin (vitamin B_2), pyridoxine (vitamin B_6), cyanocobalamin (vitamin B_{12}), tocopherol (vitamin E), carotenoids, and tryptophan in Thai women using OCs. The only significant findings were elevated vitamin A and folic acid in serum and red blood cells (Ref 7).

Because OCs decrease serum levels of folic acid and because pregnancy increases the body's requirement of it, women who become pregnant shortly after discontinuing OCs may have greater chances of developing folate deficiency and its complications. All women, regardless of OC use, should begin taking neonatal vitamins containing 1 mg folic acid three months prior to attempting to become pregnant in order to decrease the risk of spina bifida and other congenital anomalies related to neural tubal defects that can result from folate deficiency.

OC users may have disturbances in normal tryptophan metabolism that may result in a relative pyridoxine deficiency. The clinical significance of this is yet to be determined.

The clinical effects of severe vitamin and mineral deficiencies are shown in Table 13. Deficiencies marked enough to cause these symptoms are rare.

Plasma levels of some nutrients (such as vitamin A, iron, and copper) increase with OC use. These increases are not substantial enough to cause clinical effects and may be beneficial for some women.

Causal Factors

Decreased intestinal absorption of vitamins and minerals causes many of the deficiencies associated with OC use. The most marked decreases are found in the water-soluble vitamins:

- Thiamine (B_1)
- Riboflavin (B_2)
- Pyridoxine (B_6)
- Cobalamin (B_{12})
- Ascorbic acid (C)
- Folacin (folic acid)

29.

Pyridoxine is utilized in the metabolism of tryptophan. Because estrogen increases tryptophan production, more pyridoxine is needed for metabolizing the increased levels of tryptophan in OC users.

Estrogen also stimulates the metabolism of vitamins, resulting in decreased levels of some vitamins, especially riboflavin (B_2), cobalamin (B_{12}), and ascorbic acid (vitamin C), in OC users. Women who smoke also have decreased levels of vitamin C. Thus, OC users who smoke may benefit from vitamin C supplements.

Because estrogen increases vitamin A carrier protein in the blood, it is thought to be responsible for the increase in this fat-soluble vitamin in OC users.

The mechanism of OC effects on zinc and magnesium is unknown.

Management

OC users who eat an adequate diet usually do not require vitamin supplementation unless they plan to become pregnant within three months (see above). Table 13 lists dietary sources of important vitamins and minerals. Women who wish to increase their intakes of vitamins and minerals can do so by increasing their intakes of these source foods rather than by taking supplements.

Vitamin and mineral increases caused by OCs do not require treatment.

References: 7, 132

WEIGHT INCREASE OR DECREASE

Clinical Information

Many studies have shown that as many women lose weight as gain weight while taking OCs. An unexpected finding in one study was that overweight women gained less weight than underweight women. Weight gain may actually be beneficial to poorly nourished women.

Causal Factors

Progestins, especially those with high androgenic activities, and estrogens can cause weight gain. Progestin- and/or androgen-induced weight gain may be due to:

- An anabolic effect, accompanied by increased appetite OR
- An altered carbohydrate metabolism, which can cause hyperinsulinemia and is accompanied by symptoms of hypoglycemia

Estrogen-induced weight gain is associated with an increase in subcutaneous fat, especially in the breasts, hips, and thighs, and is not accompanied by increased appetite.

Weight gain may also be associated with fluid retention due to either component of the OC. This type of weight gain is cyclic and is usually accompanied by other symptoms of fluid retention.

Management

OCs with lower progestational/androgenic activities may be of benefit if weight gain is accompanied by:
- Increased appetite
- Symptoms of hypoglycemia

A diet designed for patients with hypoglycemia and caloric reduction will reduce weight gain due to a progestational effect or from other causes.

OCs with lower estrogenic activities may be of benefit if the weight gain:
- Occurs mainly in the breasts, hips, and thighs
- Is cyclic
- Is accompanied by bloating or edema

References: 7, 83, 180, 419, 498

DIETARY AND EXERCISE AMENORRHEA

Dietary and exercise amenorrhea will produce low test results on levels of:
- Follicle stimulating hormone (FSH)
- Prolactin
- Thyroid hormones

Careful histories and analyses of patients usually reveal total daily caloric intakes of less than 1,000 and carbohydrate intakes of less than 100 grams. Glucose tolerance tests (GTTs) performed on patients with dietary amenorrhea will commonly be flat (i.e., return to fasting levels one hour after the glucose challenge).

Dietary amenorrhea is often resistant to most forms of medical treatment, including ovarian stimulation with menopausal gonadotropins, but menses will resume after food intake is increased to 1,800 calories per day with at least 200 grams of carbohydrate.

If amenorrhea is due to excessive exercise, FSH and thyroid levels will be low normal and prolactin levels may initially be slightly elevated. Menses may resume when caloric intake is increased and/or exercise is decreased.

CHANGES IN LABORATORY VALUES

Interactions with Laboratory Tests

Certain endocrine and liver function tests and blood components may be affected by oral contraceptives:

- Increased prothrombin and factors VII, VIII, IX, and X; decreased antithrombin 3; and increased norepinephrine-induced platelet aggregability
- Increased thyroid-binding globulin (TBG) leading to increased circulating total thyroid hormone, as measured by protein-bound iodine (PBI), T_4 by column or by radioimmunoassay. Free T_3 resin uptake is decreased, reflecting the elevated TBG. Free T_4 concentration is altered
- Other binding proteins may be elevated in serum
- Sex steroid binding globulins are increased and result in elevated levels of total circulating sex steroids and corticoids; however, free or biologically-active levels remain unchanged
- Triglycerides may be increased
- Glucose tolerance may be decreased
- Serum folate levels may be depressed by oral contraceptive therapy. This may be of clinical significance if a woman becomes pregnant shortly after discontinuing oral contraceptives

-FDA Package Insert Labeling

OCs cause a number of laboratory changes, most of which are related to the estrogen component (Table 10).

References: 83, 109

NOTES

#30 Musculoskeletal System

Leg Pain, Cramps, and Swelling
Rheumatoid Arthritis
Muscle Function
Bone Mass

LEG PAIN, CRAMPS, AND SWELLING

Clinical Information

Bilateral leg cramps and swelling of the lower extremities often disappear spontaneously after the third cycle of OC use. Leg cramps are also noted with danazol use.

Unilateral leg swelling may be due to thrombophlebitis or thrombosis. Signs of thrombosis include:

- An increase in size and warmth of the leg
- Pain on palpation and dorsiflexion of the foot (Homan's sign)
- A palpable cord
- The presence of varicosities

A rapid increase in pain over a 24-hour period also indicates probable thrombosis as a cause. Preceding the onset of symptoms, patients may have experienced an incidence of:

- Recent injury
- Immobilization
- Sitting for prolonged periods

Pain in the chest and/or shortness of breath may indicate that a pulmonary embolus has occurred.

Causal Factors

Bilateral leg pain may be insignificant and the result of fluid retention, especially if accompanied by cramps. Fluid retention that is due to OC use may result from either the estrogen or the progestin/androgen component of the OC. Leg cramps are common in women who take danazol for treatment of endometriosis.

Bilateral leg pain may also result from venous dilatation due to the smooth muscle relaxing effect of progestin.

Unilateral leg pain may be the result of thrombophlebitis or thrombosis and requires careful evaluation.

Management

In all cases of leg pain, an examination must be performed to rule out thrombosis.

If thrombosis is suspected, OCs should be stopped until the cause of pain is determined. A diagnosis of thrombosis or thromboembolism is an absolute contraindication to further OC use (see Section #12).

Bilateral swelling due to fluid retention may be relieved by a switch in OCs to one with lower estrogenic or androgenic activity. A low-sodium diet may reduce edema in some cases.

Bilateral leg pain associated with venous dilatation and varicose veins but not thrombosis or thrombophlebitis may be relieved by a switch in OCs to one with lower progestational activity. Bilateral leg cramps may also be relieved by an increase in calcium intake.

If swelling and pain persist, an alternative method of birth control should be considered.

References: 81, 83

RHEUMATOID ARTHRITIS

Rheumatoid arthritis may be reduced by OC use. In two studies, the risk of rheumatoid arthritis in OC users was 49 percent and the risk in women who had ever used OCs was 42 percent of that of nonusers. There has been a decline in the incidence of rheumatoid arthritis in women but not in men in the U.S. since 1964. Additionally, studies involving smaller numbers of patients have been unable to confirm a protective effect against rheumatoid arthritis in OC users or former users.

30.

References: 5, 8, 9, 79, 141, 237, 242, 359, 360, 445, 446

MUSCLE FUNCTION

OCs do not enhance athletic performance as has been noted with danazol (used for treatment of endometriosis). Specifically, OCs do not affect ventilatory response to treadmill exercise or change post-exercise muscle lactate or glycogen but do decrease grip endurance times.

References: 141, 483

BONE MASS

OCs increase vertebral bone calcium by about one percent per year of use in young and premenopausal women. No increase in peripheral skeletal bone mass was noted in two studies, although radius bone mass increased with high-estrogen OCs and bone calcium turnover was retarded with a moderately androgenic OC.

References: 58, 141, 240, 340

NOTES

#31 Neuropsychological System

Depression
Emotional Changes
Libido Changes
Psychiatric Disorders
Epilepsy

Emotional Disorders
   Women with a history of depression should be carefully observed and the drug (OCs) discontinued if depression recurs to a serious degree.

-FDA Package Insert Labeling

DEPRESSION

Clinical Information
   Depression is a condition marked by:
- Apathy
- Listlessness
- Feelings of dejection
- Loss of appetite
- Insomnia
- Restlessness
- Tiredness
- Fatigue
- Weakness

Causal Factors
   Patients taking phenothiazines or tricyclic antidepressants may be hypoestrogenic or anovulatory because of decreased gonadotropin levels. OCs may ameliorate the effects of low estrogen or progesterone.
   Symptoms of tiredness and weakness in OC users may be due to the progestin component and are similar to symptoms due to increased progesterone in mid- and late pregnancy.
   Such symptoms may also occur due to low blood sugar (hypoglycemia) or hypothyroidism. Clinicians should investigate these conditions before they switch patients to OCs with different progestin doses.

Chronic tiredness may also be the result of:
- Chronic poor health
- Malnutrition caused by inadequate or "fad" diets
- Severe anemia
- Pregnancy

Some symptoms may be due to vitamin B_6 (pyridoxine) deficiency.

Management

Patients with histories of psychic depression should be carefully observed and OCs discontinued if the depression recurs during OC use.

The possible enhanced hepatic metabolism of contraceptive steroids induced by antiseizure medications must be considered (see Tables 14 and 15). Alternatively, use of other types of antidepressants may be considered. (Patients requiring drugs listed in Table 14 may require higher doses of OCs or may need to use other methods of contraception.)

Switching patients to OCs with lower progestin doses will relieve symptoms of tiredness in depression cases not due to organic causes (Table 5).

References: 109, 110, 356, 466, 498

EMOTIONAL CHANGES

Clinical Information

Emotional changes may include:
- Easily excited or agitated emotions
- Feelings of unrest
- Irritability

31.

If these symptoms occur during the 21 days in which active OCs are taken and are accompanied by fluid retention, they are usually due to estrogen excess.

If nervousness and irritability occur without accompanying symptoms of estrogen excess or edema during the days that active OCs are taken, the symptoms may be due to low estrogenic activity or hypoglycemia.

Causal Factors

Emotional upset often occurs premenstrually in ovulatory women. Symptoms may be part of the premenstrual fluid-retention syndrome caused by sodium and water retention. Depending on their associations with fluid retention, these symptoms may be the result of either excessive or insufficient estrogenic activity in OCs. Symptoms may also be due to low blood glucose levels.

Irritability associated with depression during OC use or after discontinuance of OCs may be due to vitamin B_6 deficiency.

Management

If symptoms are relieved by sugar intake, patients have hypoglycemia or possibly diabetes. If the diagnosis of hypoglycemia is confirmed, patients should be advised to eat low-sugar/high-protein diets and switched to OCs with lower progestational and androgenic activities (Table 5).

If nervousness and irritability occur both during the days active OCs are taken and during pill-free days or if they occur without accompanying edema at any time, patients should be switched to OCs with greater estrogenic activities that do not exceed 35 mcg of estrogen. (Table 5 lists relative estrogenic activities of different OCs.)

If irritability is accompanied by edema during the days active OCs are taken, patients should be switched to OCs with lower estrogenic activities.

Monophasic OCs may be helpful for patients with mood swings.

Vitamin B_6 may be helpful, especially with accompanying depression.

References: 83, 498

LIBIDO CHANGES

Clinical Information

The libido may be identified variously as:

- Sex drive
- Sexual feelings
- Sexual nature

A statistically significant decrease in libido has been reported in some OC users.

An increase in libido has also been suggested to occur in some women.

Causal Factors

The libido is related to the effective amount of testosterone in the blood, most of which is bound to sex hormone binding gonadotropin (SHBG). A decrease in libido may be due to:

- Suppression of ovarian testosterone production due to OC activity
- A direct action on the brain by estrogen or progestin
- An increase in SHBG induced by estrogens

Decreased sexual feelings occur most often with high-progestin/high-estrogen OCs.

An increase in libido may result from:

- A decrease in SHBG (resulting in an increase of free testosterone)
- Inherent androgenic effects of some progestins (see Section #15)
- Reduced anxiety about becoming pregnant

Management

If decreased libido occurs, patients should be switched to OCs with lower estrogenic and progestational activities or with higher androgenic activities.

If increased libido occurs and is a problem, patients should be switched to OCs with lower androgenic activities and higher estrogenic and progestational activities, such as those containing ethynodiol diacetate.

References: 83, 356

PSYCHIATRIC DISORDERS

Clinical Information

Despite occasional case reports, large controlled studies have shown no difference between OC users and nonusers in incidences of:

- Schizophrenia
- Anxiety
- Hysterical neuroses
- Obsessive states
- Nervous breakdowns
- Psychogenic gastrointestinal problems
- Sleep disorders
- Situational disturbances

The incidence of phobic neuroses is decreased with OC use, but this is believed to be due to self-selection by the patient.

One study found no increase in the incidence of serious psychiatric illness as measured by first referral to a hospital among 9,504 OC users compared to diaphragm and intrauterine device (IUD) users.

In institutionalized patients accustomed to long-term drug regimens, compliance is high and OCs are an appropriate choice in the absence of risk factors. Compliance is difficult to ensure in outpatients; thus, implants, injections, or IUDs may offer better contraception for these patients (Ref 161). The availability of long-acting implants and steroid contraception makes sterilization unnecessary except in rare circumstances.

Reference: 161, 356

EPILEPSY

Not all seizures are due to epilepsy; therefore, a definitive diagnosis of recurrent epilepsy should be established before altering contraceptive treatment.

Approximately one percent of the population has epilepsy (Ref 165). Clinical studies have not demonstrated exacerbation of epileptic seizures by OCs (Ref 260). The major concern is that anti-epileptic drugs, many of which are teratogenic, decrease steroid concentration and, therefore, effectiveness of some OCs (Ref 72). Serum levels of progesterone are not affected by anti-epileptic drugs as much as levels of estrogen. Progesterone appears to inhibit seizures.

Epileptic seizures tend to occur shortly preceding menses. Seizures occur more frequently during anovulatory cycles than ovulatory cycles (Ref 258). Progesterone decreases and estrogen increases electroencephalogram (EEG) spikes (Ref 11). Intramuscular (IM) medroxyprogesterone acetate (MPA) has been shown to decrease the number of seizures (Ref 259).

Many anticonvulsant drugs induce metabolism of ethinyl estradiol and lower plasma concentrations of estrogen, thereby increasing the risk of breakthrough bleeding and pregnancy (see Table 14). The exception is valproic acid.

Management

It is important that women with epilepsy use higher-dose progestins, although 30 to 35 mcg estrogen should be sufficient (not the 50 mcg estrogen OCs, as suggested by some authors). IM MPA may also be used, but implants may not be effective. Valproic acid does not induce hepatic enzymes and is the drug of choice for epileptic women who need contraception; however, it is associated with an increased risk of spina bifida.

Reference: 11, 72, 165, 258, 259, 260, 261, 356, 375

#32 Neurosensory System

Headache
Migraine
Dizziness
Hot Flushes/Hot Feelings
Numbness or Tingling of Extremities
Vision Changes
Hearing Changes
Sense of Smell
Sense of Taste

Sensory/nervous system symptoms are often difficult to assess. Although many of these symptoms are unrelated to OC use, some that appear after OCs are begun are of a potentially serious nature and require immediate attention.

HEADACHE

General Information
Headaches are one of the most common patient complaints and occur more frequently in women than in men. They may be a manifestation of body conditions or disease processes. Most occur in the absence of organic pathological conditions, but some may be associated with serious illness.

Types of headaches
Headaches due to fluid retention
Headaches due to fluid retention are usually associated with:
- Edema of the legs
- Bloating
- Breast tenderness
- Weight gain

Tension Headaches
Tension headaches are commonly characterized as:
- Gradually increasing in intensity
- Nonthrobbing

- Generally occurring bilaterally in the back of the head and neck
- Occasionally occurring bilaterally and at the temples

Migrane or vascular headaches

Migraine or vascular headaches are characterized as:

- Occurring unilaterally
- Progressive in intensity
- Throbbing at their height
- Sometimes associated with a transient prodrome of:
  - Nausea
  - Dizziness
  - Scintillating scotoma (flashing lights)
  - Numbness of an arm or leg

In rare cases, increased headaches are a warning sign of hypertension.

Tension headaches are a common occurrence. Most are benign and unrelated to OC use.

Fluid retention headaches and vascular spasm (migraine) may be related to OC use. Both types are believed to be due to estrogen.

MIGRAINE

> The onset or exacerbation of migraine or development of headache with a new pattern which is recurrent, persistent, or severe requires discontinuance of oral contraceptives and evaluation of the cause.
>
> *-FDA Package Insert Labeling*

Approximately 18 percent of women and six percent of men have one or more migraine headaches each year. The prevalence in both men and women is highest between ages 35 and 45 (Ref 403). Increase in migraine headaches during menses is reported by 55 percent of women (Ref 285). By contrast, 75 percent of migraine patients report no headaches during pregnancy, and 47 percent note a worsening of headaches after menopause.

An early case control study found the risk of thrombotic stroke was increased twofold in migraine

32.

patients who did not use OCs and 5.9 times in OC users (Ref 64). This study has never been confirmed.

The Walnut Creek study was unable to demonstrate a higher incidence of migraine in OC patients (Ref 361). Another early study found migraine headaches more severe but not more frequent in OC users. It also found headaches concentrated in pill-free days and the first days of a new pill cycle (Ref 131). Premenstrual administration of estrogen prevents the onset of migraine (Ref 74). Thus, the bulk of evidence suggests that withdrawal from estrogen at the time of menses leads to migraine (Ref 261).

As many as one-third of migraine patients note improvement in their conditions when using OCs (Ref 261). In contrast, patients who have new onset of migraine-type vascular headaches during OC use do not have attacks during the pill-free intervals (Ref 136). Estrogen implants improved migraine conditions in 96 percent of women, and 80 percent became completely or almost completely headache-free (Ref 74, 411).

Thrombotic stroke seems to be more common in OC users who first experience migraines while taking OCs than in women who have migraines before using OCs (Ref 261). Headaches can be a warning sign of cerebral thrombosis. Cerebral thrombosis-associated headaches are often but are not necessarily of the migraine type and may be due to vascular spasm. The majority of OC users who develop strokes (cerebral vascular accidents [CVAs]) experience headaches for weeks or months before the CVA event.

Management

OCs may be an appropriate choice of contraception for women with pre-existing migraine that does not worsen while taking OCs. However, such women should be monitored closely for an increase in severity or frequency of headaches.

Women who first experience migraine or focal neurological symptoms while taking OCs or who note worsening of pre-existing headaches should stop OC use immediately and substitute other methods of contraception.

Clinicians should recommend alternative contraceptive methods for these patients and may wish to discuss permanent birth control with patients who have achieved their desired family size.

If headaches are clearly associated with fluid excess, patients should be switched to OCs with lower estrogenic activities (Table 5). If headaches persist after switching OCs, patients should discontinue OCs and use alternative contraceptive methods.

References: 73, 74, 83, 87, 109, 110, 131, 136, 261, 285, 330, 331, 356, 361, 403, 411

DIZZINESS

Clinical Information

Dizziness may be described as:
- Lightheadedness
- Faintness
- Syncope
- Vertigo

Dizziness often occurs in association with fluid retention and usually disappears after the third cycle of OC use. It may also be due to low blood pressure (hypotension) or severe anemia.

Dizziness that occurs two to four hours after a meal that has a high carbohydrate content may be due to hypoglycemia. Symptoms of hypoglycemia are believed to be due to the progestin component of OCs (see Section #13).

Causal Factors

Although its exact etiology is unknown, dizziness is common in early pregnancy and may be related to estrogen.

Management

Patients who are well informed about the potential side effect of dizziness seem to adjust better than those who are not. If symptoms persist after the third cycle of OC use, patients may be switched to OCs with lower estrogenic activities. If no relief occurs, other causes of dizziness should be explored.

If symptoms are believed to be due to hypoglycemia, patients should be:

- Switched to OCs with lower progestational activities and advised to eat low-carbohydrate diets OR
- Advised to use alternative contraceptive methods (Table 2)

References: 83, 501

HOT FLUSHES/HOT FEELINGS

Clinical Information

Hot flushes are uncommon in OC users because OCs, even those with less than 50 mcg estrogen, have estrogenic activities equal to or greater than doses used for menopausal replacement.

Hot flushes occurring during the seven days that active OCs are not taken may signal that a woman has reached menopause and no longer needs OCs.

Causal Factors

Hot flushes or hot feelings experienced by some OC users are probably due to the thermogenic effect of progestin. The temperature increase caused by progestins is no greater than that occurring during pregnancy and is not serious or harmful.

These symptoms are frequent complaints of women in countries that have warm climates, because of the combined effects of the climates and progestin.

Hot flushes common during menopause are a vascular effect due to low estrogen or high luteinizing hormone (LH) levels.

Localized heat in an extremity may be due to thrombosis (see Section #12).

Management

If hot flushes occur during OC use, patients should be switched to OCs with greater estrogenic activities if no contraindications are present.

If hot flushes occur during the seven days that active OCs are not taken and patients are believed to be near menopause, OCs may be discontinued and progestin-only OCs or other contraceptive methods used for a six-month period. If no menses occur during this time, the patient is probably menopausal and contraceptive efforts may be discontinued. If galactorrhea is present, however, patients should be evaluated for possible accompanying amenorrhea (see Section #28).

Most symptoms of hot feelings require no treatment, although switching patients to lower progestin dose OCs may be helpful.

References: 83, 89

NUMBNESS OR TINGLING OF EXTREMITIES

Clinical Information

Numbness or tingling of extremities may be described as:

- A pins and needles feeling
- Unilateral or bilateral paralysis
- Weakness of an extremity

Unilateral weakness or paralysis commonly occurs preceding migraine attack. The risk of cerebral thrombosis appears to be increased in women with unilateral symptoms.

Symptoms of numbness or tingling are usually transient and are relieved after OC use is discontinued.

Causal Factors

These symptoms may signify cerebral vascular spasm if they are unilateral and involve both upper and lower extremities. If bilateral, symptoms may be due to simple fluid retention.

Management

If unilateral symptoms occur, OCs must be discontinued and alternative contraceptive methods used.

Bilateral symptoms of a mild nature may be managed by switching patients to OCs with lower estrogenic activities. If bilateral symptoms persist, OCs should be permanently discontinued.

VISION CHANGES

Ocular Lesions

There have been clinical case reports of retinal thrombosis associated with the use of oral contraceptives. Oral contraceptives should be discontinued if there is unexplained partial or complete loss of vision, onset of proptosis or diplopia, papilledema, or retinal vascular lesions. Appropriate diagnostic and therapeutic measures should be undertaken immediately.

Contact Lenses

Contact lens wearers who develop visual changes or changes in lens tolerance should be assessed by an ophthalmologist.

-FDA Package Insert Labeling

Clinical Information

Vision changes may be characterized as:
- Blurring of vision
- Scintillating scotoma
- Diplopia
- Papilledema
- Difficulty with refraction of lens
- Proptosis
- Sudden diminished vision
- Sudden loss of vision

These visual symptoms are generally regarded as serious. They may be related to OC use (as have reported neuroocular lesions, such as optic neuritis and retinal artery thrombosis).

Visual symptoms due to vascular spasm that may precede stroke are:
- Scintillating scotoma
- Proptosis
- Sudden diminished vision
- Transient loss of sight

Causal Factors

High levels of estrogen, as occur during pregnancy and sometimes during OC use, cause swelling of the cornea and changes of its curvature. This results in vision changes.

Management

Funduscopic examination is essential in diagnosing vision changes. A blurring of vision due to edema needs to be differentiated from changes due to vascular spasm.

If patients have difficulty with refraction, they should be switched to OCs with lower estrogenic activities (Table 5).

Patients should discontinue OC use immediately and consult their physicians if they experience symptoms of:

- Vascular spasm
- Sudden onset of diplopia
- Sudden/gradual or partial/complete loss of vision
- Sudden onset of papilledema
- Retinal vascular lesions

Clinicians should institute appropriate diagnostic and therapeutic measures for these patients and counsel them to use alternative contraceptive methods.

Some ophthalmologists recommend that women who develop retinitis pigmentosa discontinue OC use, since estrogen may accelerate peripheral field loss, as occurs in pregnancy.

References: 109, 110, 330, 331

HEARING CHANGES

Hearing changes are not believed to be due to OC use. Reduction of ear wax is the only known effect of OCs on hearing, and this is believed to be due to an estrogenic effect of reducing sebum secretion.

SENSE OF SMELL

The sense of smell is not known to be affected by OC use; but, with increasing doses of estrogen, there is a corresponding increase in:
- Nasal catarrh
- Hay fever
- Allergic rhinitis
- Nasal polyps

SENSE OF TASTE

Taste is sometimes reported to be affected by OC use. Some OC users and some pregnant women report an unpleasant sweet taste in the mouth. OC users may have increased incidences of:
- Salivary calculi
- Gingivitis
- Mouth ulcers

No effect on the tongue is known.

NOTES

#33 Respiratory/Urinary Systems

Respiratory Infections
Chest Pain/Shortness of Breath
Cystic Fibrosis
Urinary Problems

RESPIRATORY INFECTIONS

Clinical Information
Acute and chronic respiratory infections appear to be increased for OC users, though the increase may be due to overreporting. There is a small but insignificant increase in the incidence of pneumonia in OC users.

OC users also have an increased incidence of:
- Acute nasopharyngitis
- Chronic nasopharyngitis
- Laryngitis
- Tracheitis
- Chronic sinusitis
- Upper respiratory infection
- Acute and chronic bronchitis

Causal Factors
Increased nasal congestion is known to occur during pregnancy, possibly due to edema and the increased vascularity of mucus membranes caused by estrogen.

Progesterone is known to be immunosuppressive, but no differences were found in the proliferative immune response of B- or T-cells in women taking low-dose OCs as compared to controls.

Management
If respiratory infections recur, patients should discontinue OC use or use OCs with reduced steroid contents.

References: 17, 280

CHEST PAIN/SHORTNESS OF BREATH

Clinical Information
A twofold increase in pleurisy was found in OC users in the Royal College of General Practitioners (RCGP) study.

Causal Factors
Causes of chest pain may include:
- Pleurisy
- Rib or cartilage trauma
- Gastritis
- Pneumonia
- Collapsed lung
- Angina

The possibility of pulmonary embolus should be suspected if chest pain is sudden in onset and is accompanied by:
- Shortness of breath
- Coughing up blood
- Concurrent or antecedent pain in an extremity
- Pain in the pelvis

Additional information on pulmonary embolism can be found in Section #12.

Management
Due to the potentially extreme seriousness of chest pain and shortness of breath, patients experiencing such symptoms should discontinue OC use and see their physicians. Patients should use alternative contraceptive methods until definite diagnosis can be made.

CYSTIC FIBROSIS

Clinical Information
One report suggested that OC use by cystic fibrosis (CF) patients may be associated with marked deterioration of pulmonary status; however, this report did not include pulmonary function studies. A prospective

33.

study of 10 adolescent and young adult OC users with moderate to severe lung disease found no significant deterioration in clinical status or pulmonary function.

Management

CF patients who use OCs should be followed carefully. These patients may experience:
- Changes in pulmonary status
- Increased incidence of polypoid cervicitis
- Increased incidence of monilia vaginitis

Reference: 92, 114

URINARY PROBLEMS

Clinical Information

Urinary problems include:
- Cystitis
- Pyelonephritis
- Urinary tract infections
- Stress incontinence (loss of urine with coughing, sneezing, or straining)

Cystitis and pyelonephritis occur significantly more often in OC users. This rate increase is related to estrogen dose.

Causal Factors

Progestational activity is partially responsible for the dilatation of ureters observed in pregnancy and may have a similar effect in OC users.

Estrogens cause hypersensitivity of the bladder and increase urinary frequency and urgency. Estrogen-caused urinary symptoms are similar to the symptoms of cystitis due to infection.

Estrogenic activity that is too low may result in:
- Uterine and bladder descensus
- Cystocele
- Stress incontinence

These symptoms may also signal the beginning of menopause if they first occur after several years of continual OC use.

Some cystitis may be related to a greater frequency of intercourse in OC users.

Management

Most cystitis is unrelated to OC use and should be treated by routine diagnostic and therapeutic methods. If cystitis occurs more frequently after OCs are started or if symptoms similar to cystitis occur without bacteria being found in the urine, patients should be switched to OCs with lower estrogenic activities, especially if other symptoms of excess estrogenic activity are present.

If loss of urine occurs and pelvic examination reveals uterine descensus that was not present before OCs were started, patients should be switched to OCs with higher estrogenic activities if no other contraindications are present.

References: 387

#34 Index

34.

Abbreviations

AFP	Alpha-fetoprotein
ASHD	Atherosclerotic heart disease
BBT	Basal body temperature
BTB	Breakthrough bleeding
CI	Confidence interval
CNS	Central nervous system
CVA	Cerebrovascular accident
CVD	Cardiovascular disease
DMPA	Depomedroxyprogesterone acetate
DS	Desogestrel
ED	Ethinodial diacetate
EE	Ethinyl estradiol
GS	Gestodene
HDL-C	High-density lipoprotein cholesterol
LDL-C	Low-density lipoprotein cholesterol
LNG	Levonorgestrel
MI	Myocardial infarction
MPA	Medroxyprogesterone actetate
NE	Norethindrone
NEA	Norethindrone acetate
NET	Norethindrone enanthanate
NG	Norgestrel
NS	Norgestimate
OC	Oral contraceptive
OR	Odds ratio
RCGP	Royal College of General Practitioners
RCOG	Royal College of Obstetrics and Gynecology
RR	Relative risk
VTE	Venous thromboembolism
WHO	World Health Organization
WYS	Women years

References

1. Abernethy DR, Greenblatt DJ, Divoll M, Arendt RL: Impairment of diazepam clearance with low-dose oral contraceptive steroid therapy. Clin Pharmacol Ther 1984;35:360-366.

2. Adam SA, Thorogood M, Mann JI: Oral contraception and myocardial infarction revisited: The effects of new preparations and prescribing patterns. Br J Obstet Gynecol 1981;88:838-845.

3. Albers JJ, Cheung MC, Hazzard WR: High-density lipoproteins in myocardial infarction survivors. Metabolism 1978;27:479.

4. Allaart CF, Poort SR, Rosendaal FR, et al.: Increased risk of venous thrombosis in carriers of hereditary protein C deficiency defect. Lancet 1993;341:134-138.

5. Allebeck P et al.: Do oral contraceptives reduce the incidence of rheumatoid arthritis? Scand J Rheumatol 1984;13:140.

6. Alpert LI: Veno-occlusive disease associated with oral contraceptives. Human Pathology 1976; 7:709-718.

7. Amatayakul K, Uttaravachai C, Singkamani R, Ruckphaopunt S: Vitamin metabolism and the effects of multivitamin supplementation in oral contraceptive users. Contraception 1984; 30(2):179-196.

8. American College of Obstetrics and Gynecologists: Oral contraception, patient counseling. ACOG Technical Bulletin, No. 41; July, 1976.

9. Andolsek L et al.: Influence of oral contraceptives on the incidence of premalignant and malignant lesions of the cervix. Contraception 1983; 28(6):505-529.

10. Arthes FC, Sartwell PE, Lewison EF: The pill, estrogens, and the breast: Epidemiological aspects. Cancer 1971;28:1391-1394.

11. Bachstrom T: Epileptic seizures in women related to plasma estrogen and progesterone during the menstrual cycle. Acta Neurol Scand 1976;54:321-347.

12. Baciewicz AM: Oral contraceptive drug interactions. Ther Drug Monit 1985;7(1):26-35.

13. Back DJ et al.: The effect of rifampicin on norethisterone pharmacokinetics. Eur J Clin Pharmacol 1971;15(3):193-197.

14. Back DJ et al.: The interaction of phenobarbital and other anticonvulsants with oral contraceptive steroid therapy. Contraception 1980;22(5):495-503.

15. Back DJ et al.: Interindividual variation and drug interactions with hormonal steroid contraceptives. Drugs 1981;21(1):46-61.

16. Back J, Grimmer SFM, Orme MLE, Proudlove C, Mann RD, et al.: Evaluation of Committee on Safety of Medicines yellow card reports on oral contraceptive drug interactions with anticonvulsants and antibiotics. Br J Clin Pharm 1988;25:527-532.

17. Baker DA, Thomas J: The effect of low-dose oral contraceptives on the initial immune response to infection. Contraception 1984;29(6):519-525.

18. Bamford PN, Forbes-Smith PA, Rose GL, et al.: An analysis of factors responsible for progression or regression of mild and moderate cervical dyskaryosis. Br J Fam Plann 1985;11:5-8.

19. Barter JF et al.: Inferior vena cava thrombosis with oral contraceptives documented by computed tomography. Obstet Gynecol 1983;61(3 Suppl):59S-62S.

20. Batzev FR: Measurement of androgenicity: The spectrum of progestogen activity. J Repro Med 1986;31(suppl):848-864.

21. Baum J et al.: Possible association between benign hepatomas and oral contraceptives. Lancet 1973;2:926-929.

22. Beck P: Effect of progestins on glucose and lipid metabolism. Ann NY Acad Sci 1977;286:434-445.
23. Beck WW Jr: Complications and contraindications of oral contraception. Clin Obstet Gynecol 1981;24:3.
24. Beller FK et al.: Effects of oral contraceptives on blood coagulation: A review. Obstet Gynecol Surv 1985;40(7):425-436.
25. Benagiano D, Primiero FM: Long-acting contraceptives: Present status. Drugs 1983;25(6):570-609.
26. Beral V, Kay CR: Mortality among oral contraceptive users. Lancet 1977;2:727-731.
27. Berenson AB, Weimann CM, Rickerr VI, McCombs SL: Contraceptive outcome among adolescents prescribed Norplant® implants vs oral contraceptives after one year of use. Am J Obstet Gynecol 1997;176:586-592.
28. Bergink EV: Binding of contraceptive progestogens to receptor proteins in human myometrium and MCF-7 cells. Br J Fam Plann 1984;10:33.
29. Berkowitz GS et al.: Oral contraceptive use and fibrocystic disease among pre- and postmenopausal women. Am J Epidemiol 1984;120(1):87-96.
30. Bibbo M et al.: Follow-up study of male and female offspring of DES-treated mothers: A preliminary report. J Repro Med 1975;15:29-32.
31. Bilotta P, Favilli S: Clinical evaluation of a monophasic ethinyl estradiol/desogestrel-containing oral contraceptive. Arzneimittel-Forschung 1988;38(II):932-934.
32. Bloemenkamp KWM, Rosendaal FR, Helmerhorst FM, Buller HR, Vandenbroucke JP: Enhancement by factor V Leiden mutation of risk of deep vein thrombosis associated with oral contraceptives containing a third-generation progestagen. Lancet 1995;346:1593-1596.

33. Blum M, Gilerovitch M, Benaim J, Appelbaum T: The correlation between chlamydia antigen, antibody, vaginal colonization, and contraceptive method in young, unmarried women. Adv Contracept 1990;6:41-45.

34. Blumenstein BA, Douglas MB, Hall WD: Blood pressure changes and oral contraceptive use: A study of 2,676 black women in the southeastern United States. Am J Epidemiol 1980;112:539-552.

35. Boston Collaborative Drug Surveillance Program. Oral contraceptives and venous thromboembolic disease, surgically-confirmed gallbladder disease, and breast tumors. Lancet 1973;1:1399-1404.

36. Boston Collaborative Drug Surveillance Program. Surgically-confirmed gallbladder disease, venous thromboembolism, and breast tumors in relation to postmenopausal estrogen therapy. N Engl J Med 1974;290:15-19.

37. Bracken MB: Oral contraception and congenital malformations in offspring: A review and meta-analysis of the prospective studies. Obstet Gynecol 1990;76(2):552-557.

38. Bradley D et al.: Serum high-density lipoprotein cholesterol in women using oral contraceptives, estrogens, and progestins. New Engl J Med 1978;299:17-20.

39. Braverman DZ et al.: Effects of pregnancy and contraceptive steroids on gallbladder function. New Engl J Med 1980;302:362.

40. Briggs MD, Briggs M: Plasma lipoprotein changes during oral contraceptives. Current Med Research and Opinion 1979;6:249.

41. Brinton LA: Oral contraceptives and cervical neoplasia. Contraception 1991;43:581-595.

42. Brinton LA et al.: Long-term use of oral contraceptives and risk of invasive cervical cancer. Int J Cancer 1986;38(3):339-344.

43. Brinton LA et al.: Risk factors for benign breast disease. Am J Epidemiol 1981;113:203-214.

44. Burslem RW: Cervical cytological screening for users of oral contraceptives. Lancet 1983;2:968.

45. Caillouette JC, Koehler AL: Phasic contraceptive pills and functional ovarian cysts. Am J Obstet Gynecol 1987;156:1538-1542.

46. Capitanio GL et al.: Lipidemic changes induced by two different oral contraception formulations. Advances in Contraception 1985;1:58.

47. Carr BR, Ory H: Estrogen and progestin components of oral contraceptives: Relationship to vascular disease. Contraception 1997;55:267-272.

48. Carr DH: Chromosome studies in selected spontaneous abortions: I. Conception after oral contraceptives. Canad Med Assoc J 1970;103:343-348.

49. CASH (NIH) Study: Oral contraceptive use and the risk of breast cancer. N Engl J Med 1985;315:405.

50. CASH Study: Stadel BV, Schlesselman JJ, Murray PA: Oral contraceptives and breast cancer. Lancet 1989;i:1257-1258.

51. CASH and NICH. Combination oral contraceptive use and the risk of endometrial cancer. JAMA 1987;257:796-800.

52. Centers for Disease Control. Oral contraceptive use and the risk of breast cancer in young women. Morbidity and Mortality Weekly Report. June 29, 1984;Vol. 33, No. 25:353-354.

53. Centers for Disease Control Cancer and Steroid Hormone Study. JAMA 1987;257(6):796-800.

54. Centers for Disease Control Cancer and Steroid Hormone Study. N Engl J Med 1986;315(7):405-411.

55. Centers for Disease Control Cancer and Steroid Hormone Study: Long-term oral contraceptive use and the risk of breast cancer. JAMA 1983;249(12):1591-1595.

56. Centers for Disease Control Cancer and Steroid Hormone Study. Oral contraceptive use and the risk of ovarian cancer. JAMA 1983;249:1596-1599.

57. Chalmers JS, Fulli-Lemaire I, Cowen PJ: Effects of the contraceptive pill on sedative responses to clonidine and apomorphine in normal women. Psych Med 1985;15:363-367.

58. Chef R: Calcium metabolism during treatment with 2.5 mg Lyndiol®, a lynestrenol-mestranol combination. Bull Soc Roy Belg Gyn Ob 1966;36:473.

59. Chihal HJW, Dickey RP, Peppler R: Estrogen potency of oral contraceptive pills. Am J Obstet Gynecol 1975;121:75-83.

60. Clavel F et al.: Breast cancer and oral contraceptives: A review. Contraception 1985;32(6):553-569.

61. Cohen CJ, Deppe G: Endometrial carcinoma and oral contraceptive pills. Am J Obstet Gynecol 1977;49:390-392.

62. Coker AL, Harlap S, Fortney JA: Oral contraceptives and reproductive cancers: Weighing the risks and benefits. Fam Plann Perspect 1993;25:17-21.

63. Collaborative Group for the Study of Stroke in Young Women. Oral contraception and increased risk of cerebral ischemia or thrombosis. N Engl J Med 1973;288:871-878.

64. Collaborative Group for the Study of Stroke in Young Women. Oral contraceptives and strokes in young women: Associated risk factors. JAMA 1975;231:718-722.

65. Collaborative Group on Hormonal Factors in Breast Cancer. Breast cancer and hormonal contraceptives: Collaborative reanalysis of individual data on 53,297 women with breast cancer and 100,239 women without breast cancer from 54 epidemiological studies. Lancet 1996;347:1713-1727.

66. Comp PC, Zacur HA: Contraceptive choices in women with coagulation disorders. Am J Obstet Gynecol 1993;168:1990-1993.

67. *Contraceptive Technology* 1990-1992, 15th ed. New York: Irvington Publishers, Inc., 1990.

68. Cook CL et al.: Pregnancy prophylaxis: Parenteral postcoital estrogen. Obstet Gynecol 1986;67:331.

69. Cook NR et al.: Regression analysis of changes in blood pressure with oral contraceptive use. Am J Epidemiol 1985;121(4):530-540.

70. Coulam CB, Annegers JF: Do anticonvulsants reduce the efficacy of oral contraceptives? Epilepsia 1979;20(5):519-525.

71. Crawford P, Chadwick D, Cleland P, Tjia J, Cowie A, et al.: The lack of effect of sodium valproate on the pharmacokinetics of oral contraceptive steroids. Contraception 1986;3:23-29.

72. Crawford P, Chadwick DJ, Martin C, Tjia J, Bach DJ, Orme M: The interaction of phenytoin and carbamazepine with combined oral contraceptive steroids. Br J Clin Pharmacol 1990;30:892-896.

73. Croft P, Hannaford PC: Risk factors for acute myocardial infarction in women: Evidence from the Royal College of General Practitioners' Oral Contraceptive Study. Br Med J 1989;298:165-168.

74. Croxatto HB, Diaz S, Robertson DN, Pavez M: Clinical chemistry in women treated with levonorgestrel implants (Norplant®) or a Tcu 200 IUD. Contraception 1983;27:281-288.

75. Cullberg G et al.: Effects of a low-dose desogestrel/ethinyl estradiol combination on hirsutism, androgens, and sex hormone-binding globulin in women with polycystic ovary syndrome. Acta Obstet Gynecol Scand 1985;64(3):195-202.

76. Darney P, Atkinson E, McPherson S, Hellerstein S, Alvarado A: Acceptance and perception of Norplant® among users in San Francisco, U.S.A. Stud Fam Plann 1990;21:152-160.

77. Davidson F et al.: The pill does not cause thrush. Br J Obstet Gynaecol 1985;92(12):1265-1266.

78. De Pirro R et al.: Changes in insulin receptors during oral contraception. J Clin Endo Metab 1981;52:29.

79. Del Junco DJ et al.: Do oral contraceptives prevent rheumatoid arthritis? JAMA 1985;254(14):1938-1941.

80. Deslypere JP, Thiery M, Vermeulen A: Effect of long-term hormonal contraception on plasma lipids. Contraception 1985;31(6):633-642.
81. Dickey RP: Diagnosis and management of patients with oral contraceptive side effects. J Cont Educ Obstet Gynecol 1978;20:19.
82. Dickey RP: Oral contraceptives: Basic considerations. In: *Human Reproduction, Conception, and Contraception*. 2nd ed. Hafez ESE (ed.) Hagerstown, PA: Harper and Row, 1978.
83. Dickey RP: The pill: Physiology, pharmacology, and clinical use. In: *Seminar in Family Planning*, 1st ed. Isenman AW, Knox EG, Tyrer L (eds.) American College of Obstetrics and Gynecology, 1972. 2nd ed., 1974.
84. Dickey RP: Treatment of post-pill amenorrhea. Int J Gynecol Obstet 1977;15:125-132.
85. Dickey RP, Berger GS: Persistent amenorrhea and galactorrhea. In: *Clinical Use of Sex Steroids*. Givens JR (ed.) Chicago: Yearbook Medical Publishing, 1980;329-388.
86. Dickey RP, Chihal HJW, Peppler R: Potency of three new low-estrogen pills. Am J Obstet Gynecol 1976;125:976-979.
87. Dickey RP, Dorr CH II: Oral contraceptives: Selection of the proper pill. Obstet Gynecol 1969;33:273.
88. Dickey RP, Stone SC: Drugs that affect the breast and lactation. Clin Obstet Gynecol 1975;18:2.
89. Dickey RP, Stone SC: Progestational potency of oral contraceptives. Am J Obstet Gynecol 1976;47:106-111.
90. Diczfalusy E: New developments in oral, injectable, and implantable contraceptives, vaginal rings, and intrauterine devices: A review. Contraception 1986;33(1):7-22.
91. Donaldson D: Male contraception: A review. J R Soc Health 1985;105(3):91-98.

92. Dooley RR, Braunstein H, Osher AB: Polypoid cervicitis in cystic fibrosis patients receiving oral contraceptives. Am J Obstet Gyencol 1974;118:971-974.

93. Duffy TJ, Ray R: Oral contraceptive use: Prospective follow-up of women with suspected glucose intolerance. Contraception 1984;30(3): 197-208.

94. Dunson TR, Amatya RN, Krueger SL: Complications and risk factors associated with the removal of Norplant® implants. Obstet Gynecol 1995;85:543-548.

95. Edelbroek PM, Zitman FG, Knoppert-van er Klein EAM, van Putten PM, de Wolff FA: Therapeutic drug monitoring of amitryptiline: Impact of age, smoking, and contraceptives on drug and metabolite levels in bulemic women. Clin Chimica Acta 1987;165:177-187.

96. Editorial: Another look at the pill and breast cancer. Lancet 1985;2(8462):985-987.

97. Editorial: Which pill? Brit Med J 1983;287:1397.

98. Edmonsen HA, Henderson B, Benton B: Liver cell adenomas associated with the use of oral contraceptives. N Engl J Med 1976;294:470-472.

99. Elam MB et al.: Mitral valve prolapse in women with oral contraceptive-related cerebrovascular insufficiency: Associated persistent hypercoagulable state. Arch Intern Med 1986;146(1):73-77.

100. Elder MG: Injectable contraception. Clin Obstet Gynaecol 1984;11(3):723-741.

101. Elger WH et al.: Endocrine pharmacological profile of gestodene. Adv Contracept Delivery Systems 1986;2:182-97.

102. Elkik F et al.: Contraception in hypertensive women using a vaginal ring delivering estradiol and levonorgestrel. J Clin Endocrinol Metab 1986;63(1):29-35.

103. Ellery C et al.: A case control study of breast cancer in relation to the use of steroid contraceptive agents. Med J Aust 1986;144(4):173-176.

104. Entrican JH, Sircus W: Chronic inflammatory bowel disease, cigarette smoking, and use of oral contraceptives (letter). Br Med J (Clin Res) 1986;292(6533):1464.

105. Fadel H et al.: Availability of norethisterone acetate from combined oral contraceptive tablets. Pharmazie 1979;34(1):49-50.

106. Farmer RDT, Lawrenson RA, Thompson CR, et al.: Population-based study of the risk of venous thromboembolism associated with low-oestrogen dose oral contraceptives. Lancet 1997;349:83-88.

107. Fasal E, Paffenbarger RS: Oral contraceptives as related to cancer and benign lesions of the breast. J Natl Cancer Inst 1975;55:767-773.

108. Fechner RE: The surgical pathology of the reproductive system and breast during oral contraceptive therapy. Pathol Ann 1971;6:299-319.

109. Federal Drug Administration Drug Bulletin. April 1990;5.

110. Federal Regulation, Title 21, Parts 310.515-516, 200-299, 300-399.

111. Ferin J: Orally-active progestational compounds. In: *International Encyclopedia of Pharmacology and Therapeutics.* Ch. 30: Human studies: Effects on the utero-vaginal tract. Sect. 48, Vol. II. Elmsford, NY: Pergamon Press, 1972.

112. Fertility and Maternal Health Drugs Advisory Committee, FDA. 1989 (Oct.).

113. Fisch IR, Freedman SH, Myatt AV: Oral contraceptives, pregnancy and blood pressure. JAMA 1972;222:1507-1509.

114. Fitzpatrick SB et al.: Use of oral contraceptives in women with cystic fibrosis. Chest 1984;86(6):863-867.

115. Ford K: Contraceptive use in the United States. Fam Plann Perspect 1978;10:264.

116. Forman D, Vincent TJ, Doll R: Cancer of the liver and the use of oral contraceptives. Br Med J 1986;292(6532):1357-1361.

117. Fotherby K: A new look at progestogens. Clin Obstet Gynecol 1984;11:701.

118. Franceschi S, Parazzini F, Negri E, et al.: Pooled analysis of three European case control studies of epithelial ovarian cancer: III. Oral contraceptive use. Int J Cancer 1991;49:61-65.

119. Franceschi S et al.: Oral contraceptives and benign breast disease: A case control study. Am J Obstet Gynecol 1984;149(6):602-606.

120. Frank P, Kay CR: Incidence of thyroid disease associated with oral contraceptives. Br Med J 1978;2:1531.

121. Fregly MJ, Thrasher TN: Response of heart rate to acute administration of isoproterenol in rats treated chronically with norethynodrel, ethinyl estradiol, and both combined. Endocrinology 1977;100(1):148-154.

122. Frick J et al.: Spermatogenesis in men treated with injections of medroxyprogesterone acetate combined with testosterone enanthate. Int J Androl 1982;5(3):246-252.

123. Friedman AJ, Thomas PP: Does low-dose combination oral contraceptive use affect uterine size or menstrual flow in premenopausal women with leiomyomas? Obstet Gynecol 1995;85:631-635.

124. Friedman CI et al.: The effect of ampicillin on oral contraceptive effectiveness. Am J Obstet Gynecol 1980;55(1):33-37.

125. Fuller JH et al.: Coronary heart disease risk and impaired glucose tolerance: The Whitehall study. Lancet 1980;1:1373.

126. Gal I, Kirman B, Stern J: Hormone pregnancy tests and congenital malformation. Nature 1967;216:83.

127. Gallagher RP et al.: Reproductive factors, oral contraceptives, and risk of malignant melanoma: Western Canada Melanoma Study. Br J Cancer 1985;52(6):901-907.

128. Gambrell RD: Incidence of breast cancer in a 22-year study of women received estrogen/progestin replacement therapy. Obstet Gynecol 1993;86:477.

129. Gambrell RD Jr: Hormones in the etiology and prevention of breast and endometrial cancer. Southern Med J 1984;77:1509-1515.

130. Gansicke A, Gansicke W, Klammt J: Effect of female sex hormones on the incidence of disordered wound healing following tooth extraction. Zahn Mund Kieferheilkd 1986;74(2):131-137.

131. Gaspard UJ, Lefebvre PJ: Clinical aspects of the relationship between oral contraceptive, abnormalities in carbohydrate metabolism, and the development of cardiovascular disease. Am J Obstet Gynecol 1990;163:334-343.

132. Geurts TBP, Goorissen EM, Sitsen JMA: *Summary of Drug Interactions with Oral Contraceptives,* Parthenon Publishing Group, Carnforth UK, New York, 1993.

133. Gill WB, Schumacher GFB, Bibbo M: Structural and functional abnormalities in the sex organs of male offsprings of mothers treated with diethylstilbestrol (DES). J Repro Med 1976;16:147-153.

134. Glasier A: Emergency postcoital contraception. New Engl J Med 1997;337:1058-1064.

135. Glasier A, Thong KJ, Dewar M et al.: Mifepristone (RU 486) compared with high-dose estrogen and progestogen for emergency postcoital contraception. 1992;327:1041-1044.

136. Godsland IF, Walton C, Felton C, Proudler A, Patel A: Insulin resistance, secretion, metabolism in users of oral contraceptives. J Clin Endocrinol Metab 1991;74:64-70.

137. Godsland IF et al.: The effects of different formulations of oral contraceptive agents on lipid and carbohydrate metabolism. N Engl J Med 1990;323:1375-1381.

138. Goldacre MJ, Loudon N, Watt B, et al.: Epidemiology and clinical significance of cervical erosion in women attending a family planning clinic. Br Med J 1978;1:748-750.

139. Goldbaum GM et al.: The relative impact of smoking and oral contraceptive use on women in the United States. JAMA 1987;258:1339.

140. Goldman EL: Estrogen OCs accelerate lupus progression. Obstet Gynecol News, 1997;14.

141. Goldzieher JW: *Hormonal Contraception: Pills, Injections and Implants*. Durant, OK: Essential Medical Information Systems, 1989.

142. Gongsakdi D, Rojanasakul A: Galactorrhea in DMPA users: Incidence and clinical significance. J Med Assoc Thai 1986;69(1):28-32.

143. Grady WR, Hayward MD, Yagi J: Contraceptive failure in the United States: Estimates from the 1982 National Survey of Family Growth. Fam Plann Perspect 1986(18); 5:200-209.

144. Graham S: Alcohol and breast cancer. N Engl J Med 1987;316:1211-1313.

145. Grant EC: Hormone balance of oral contraceptives. J Obstet Gynecol 1967;74:908-918.

146. Gray RH: Toxic shock syndrome and oral contraception. Am J Obst Gynecol 1988;156:1038.

147. Gray RH, Pardthaisong T: Utero exposure to steroid contraceptives and survival during infancy. Am J Epidermiol. 1991;134:795-803.

148. Green A, Bain C: Hormonal factors and melanoma in women. Med J Aust 1985;142(8):446-448.

149. Greenblatt RB: Progestational agents in clinical practice. Med Sci 1967;5:37-49.

150. Greene GR, Sartwell PE: Oral contraceptive use in patients with thromboembolism following surgery, trauma or infection. Am J Pub Health 1972;62:680-685.

151. Greenwald P et al.: Vaginal cancer after maternal treatment with synthetic estrogens. N Engl J Med 1971;285:390-392.

152. Grimes DA, Godwin AJ, Rubin A, Smith JA, Lacarra M: Ovulation and follicular development associated with three low-dose oral contraceptives: A randomized controlled trial. Obstet Gynecol 1994;83:29-34.

153. Grimmer SFM, Allen WL, Back DJ, Breckenridge AM, Orme M, et al.: The effect of cotrimoxazole on oral contraceptive steroids in women. Contraception 1983;28:53-59.

154. Gringras M, Beaumont G, Grieve A: Clomipramine and oral contraceptives: An interaction study: Clinical findings. J Int Med Res 1980;3:76-80.

155. Grundy SM et al.: The place of HDL in cholesterol management: A perspective from the National Cholesterol Education Program. Arch Intern Med 1989;149:505-510.

156. Guillebaud J: Epidemiology of endometriosis. Letter to the editor. Br Med J 1993;306:931.

157. Gurpide E: Antiestrogenic actions of progesterone and progestins in women. In: *Progesterone and Progestins.* Bardin CW, Milgrom E, Mauvais-Jarvis P (eds.) New York: Raven Press, 1983;149-161.

158. Haber I, Hubens H: Cholestatic jaundice after triacetyloleandomycin and oral contraceptives. Acta Gastro-Enterol Belgica 1980;43:475.

159. Hammerstein J, Daume E, Simon A, et al.: Influences of gestodene and desogestrel components of low-dose oral contraceptives on the pharmacokinetics and ethinyl estradiol on serum CBG and on urinary cortisol and 6ß-hydroxycortisol. Contraception 1993;47:263-281.

160. Hannaford PC, Croft PR, Kay CR: Oral contraception and stroke: Evidence from the Royal College of General Practitioners' Oral Contraception Study. Stroke 1994;25:935-942.

161. Hankoff LD, Darney PD: Contraceptive choices for behaviorally disordered women. Am J Obstet Gynecol 1993;168:1986-1989.

162. Harlap S, Baras M: Conception waits in fertile women after stopping oral contraceptives. Int J Fertil 1984;29(2):73-80.

163. Harlap S, Shino PH, Ramcharan S: Congenital abnormalities in the offspring of women who used oral and other contraceptives around the time of conception. Int J Fertil 1985;30(2):39-47.

164. Harlap S et al.: Chromosomal abnormalities in the Kaiser-Permanente Birth Defects Study, with special reference to contraceptive use around the time of conception. Teratology 1985;31(3):381-387.

165. Hauser WA, Hesdorffer DC: Epilepsy: *Frequency, Causes, and Consequences.* New York: Demos Publications, 1990.

166. Heinermann LAJ, Lewis MA, Thorogood M, Spitzer WO, Guggenmoos-Holzmann I, Bruppacher R: Case control study of oral contraceptives and risk of thromboembolis stroke: Results from international study on oral contraceptives and health of young women. Br Med J 1997;315:1502-1504.

167. Heinonen OP et al.: Cardiovascular birth defects and antenatal exposure to female sex hormones. N Engl J Med 1977;296:67-70.

168. Heintz APM, Hacker NF, Lagasse LD: Epidemiology and etiology of ovarian cancer: A review. Obstet Gynecol 1985;66:127-135.

169. Helmrich SP et al.: Lack of an elevated risk of malignant melanoma in relation to oral contraceptive use. J N Clin 1984;72(3):617-620.

170. Henderson BE, Ross RK, Pike MC: Hormonal chemoprevention of cancer in women. Science 1993;259:633-638.

171. Henderson BE et al.: Urogenital tract abnormalities in sons of women treated with diethylstilbestrol. Pediatrics 1976;58:505-507.

172. Hennekens CH et al.: A case-control study of oral contraceptive use and breast cancer. J N Clin 1984;72(1):39-42.

173. Herbst AL, Berek JS: Impact of contraception on gynecologic cancers. Am J Obstet Gynecol 1993;168:1980-1985.

174. Herbst AL, Kurman RJ, Scully RE: Vaginal and cervical abnormalities after exposure to stilbestrol *in utero.* Obstet Gynecol 1972;40:287-298.

175. Herbst AL, Ulfedler H, Poskanzer DC: Adenocarcinoma of the vagina. N Engl J Med 1971;284:878-881.

176. Heloffspring with unexposed controls. N Engl J Med 1975;292:334-339.

179. Hislop TG, Threlfall WJ: Oral contraceptives and benign breast disease. Am J Epidemiol 1984;120(2):273-280.

180. Hjelt K et al.: Oral contraceptives and the cobalamin (vitamin B_{12}) metabolism. Acta Obstet Gynecol Scand 1985;64(1):59-63.

181. Ho PC, Kwan MSW: A prospective randomized comparison of levonorgestrel with Yuzpe regimen in postcoital contraception. Human Repro 1993;(8)3:389-392.

182. Hoyle M et al.: Small bowel ischaemia and infarction in young women taking oral contraceptives and progestational agents. Br Med J 1977;64:533.

183. Huggins GR, Guintoli RL: Oral contraceptives and neoplasia. Fertil Steril 1979;32:1.

184. Huggins GR, Zucker PK: Oral contraceptives and neoplasia. Fertil Steril 1987;47:733.

185. Hull VJ: The effects of hormonal contraceptives on lactation: Current findings, methodological considerations, and future priorities. Stud Fam Plann 1981;12(4):134-155.

186. Inman WHW, Vessey MP: Investigation of deaths from pulmonary, coronary, and cerebral thrombosis and embolism in women of childbearing age. Br Med J 1968;2:193-199.

187. Inman WHW et al.: Thromboembolic disease and the steroidal content of oral contraceptives: A report to the Committee on Safety of Drugs. Br Med J 1970;2:203-209.

188. Irey NS, Norris HJ: Intimal vascular lesions associated with female reproductive steroids. Arch Pathol Lab Med 1973;96:227-234.

189. Jacobs MB: Hepatic infarction related to oral contraceptive use. Arch Intern Med 1984;144(3):642-643.
190. Jain AK: Mortality risk associated with the use of oral contraceptives. Stud Fam Plann 1977;8:50-54.
191. Janerich DT, Piper JM, Glebatis DM: Oral contraceptives and congenital limb-reduction defects. N Engl J Med 1974;291:697-700.
192. Jensen G, Nyboe J, Appleyard M, Schnohr P: Risk factors for acute myocardial infarction in Copenhagen. II: Smoking, alcohol intake, physical activity, obesity, oral contraception, diabetes, lipids, and blood pressure. Eur Heart 1991;12:298-308.
193. Jick H, Jick SS, Gurewich V, Myers MW, Vasilakis C: Risk of ideopathic cardiovascular death and nonfatal venous thromboembolism in women using oral contraceptives with differing progestogen components. Lancet 1995;346:1589-1593.
194. Jick H, Jick SS, Meyers MW, Vasilakis C: Risk of acute myocardial infarction and low-dose combined oral contraceptives. Lancet 1996;347:627-628.
195. Jick SS, Walker AM, Jick H: Oral contraceptives and endometrial cancer. Obstet Gynecol 1993;82:931-935.
196. Jimenez J et al.: Long-term follow-up of children breastfed by mothers receiving depo-medroxyprogesterone acetate. Contraception 1984;30(6):523-533.
197. Jones RC, Edgren RA: The effects of various steroids on vaginal histology in the rat. Fertil Steril 1973;24:284-291.
198. Joshi JV et al.: A study of interaction of a low-dose combination oral contraceptive with ampicillin and metronidazole. Contraception 1980;22(6):643-652.
199. Joshi JV et al.: A study of interaction of a low-dose combination oral contraceptive with antitubercular drugs. Contraception 1980;21(6):617-629.

200. Josimovich JB et al.: Heterogeneous distribution of serum prolactin values in apparently healthy young women and the effects of oral contraceptive medication. Fertil Steril 1987;47:785.

201. Jung-Hoffmann C, Kuhl J: Interaction with the pharmacokinetics of ethinyl estradiol and progestogens contained in oral contraceptives. Contraception 1989;40:299-312.

202. Kalache A, Vessey MP: Risks factors for breast cancer. In: *Breast Cancer: Clinics of Oncology.* Baum M (ed.) Philadelphia: WB Saunders, 1982.

203. Kalkoff RW: Effect of oral contraceptive agents and sex steroids on carbohydrate metabolism. Ann Rev Med 1972;23:429-438.

204. Kasan PN, Andrews J: The effects of recent oral contraceptive use on the outcome of pregnancy. Eur J Obstet Gynecol Reprod Biol 1986;22(1-2):77-83.

205. Kaufman DW et al.: Decreased risk of endometrial cancer among oral contraceptive users. N Engl J Med 1980;303:1045.

206. Kay CR: Oral communication. Royal Society of Medicus Meeting on Oral Contraceptives and Breast Cancer, July 17-19, 1989.

207. Kay CR: Oral contraceptives and cancer. Lancet 1983;2:1018-1021.

208. Kay CR: Personal communication.

209. Kay CR: Progestogens before and after menopause. Br Med J 1980;281:811-812.

210. Kendall MJ, Jack DB, Quarterman CP, Smith SR, Zaman R: ß-andrenoceptor blocker pharmacokinetics and the oral contraceptive pill. Br J Clin Phar 1984;17:87S-89S.

211. Kennedy KI, Short RV, Tully MR: Premature introduction of progestin-only contraceptive methods during lactation. Contraception 1997;347-350.

212. Khoo SK: Cancer risks and the contraceptive pill: What is the evidence after nearly 25 years of use? Med J Auth 1986;144(4):185-190.

213. Kjaeldgaard A, Larsson B: Long-term treatment with combined oral contraceptives and cigarette smoking associated with impaired activity of tissue plasminogen activator. Acta Obstet Gynecol Scand 1996;65:219-222.

214. Kloosterboer HJ, Deckers GHJ: Desogestrel: A selective progestogen. Int Proc J 1989;1:26-30.

215. Kloosterboer HJ, Vonk-Noordegraaf CA, Turpijn EW: Selectivity in progesterone and androgen receptor binding of progestins used in oral contraceptives. Contraception 1988;38:325-32.

216. Klove KL, Roy S, Lobo RA: The effect of different contraceptive treatments on the serum concentration of dehydroepiandrosterone sulfate. Contraception 1984;29(4):319-324.

217. Knopp RH: Arteriosclerosis risk: The roles of oral contraceptives and postmenopausal estrogens. J Reprod Med 1986;31(9 Suppl):913-921.

218. Knopp RH, LaRosa JC, Burkman RT: Contraception and dyslipidemia. Am J Obstet Gynecol 1993;168-1994-2005.

219. Knopp RH et al.: Oral contraceptive and postmenopausal estrogen effects on lipoprotein, triglyceride, and cholesterol in an adult female population: Relationships to estrogen and progestin potency. J Clin Endocrinol Metab 1981;53:1123.

220. Krauss RM et al.: Effects of two low-dose oral contraceptives on serum lipids and lipoproteins: Differential changes in high-density lipoprotein subclasses. Am J Obstet Gynecol 1983;145:446-452.

221. Krettek JE, Arkin SI et al.: *Chlamydia trachomatis* in patients who used oral contraceptives and had intermenstrual spotting. Obstet and Gynecol 1993;81:728-731.

222. Kubba AAC, Guillebud J: Case of ectopic pregnancy after postcoital contraception with ethinyl oestradiol-levonorgestrel. Br Med J 1983;287:1343.

223. Kuenssberg EV et al.: Recommendations from the findings by the RCGP oral contraception study on the mortality risk of oral contraceptive users. Br Med J 1977;2:947.

224. Kung AW, Ma JT, Wong VC, et al.: Glucose and lipid metabolism with triphasic oral contraceptives in women with history of gestational diabetes. Contraception 1987;35:257-269.

225. Kunin CM, McCormack RC, Abernathy JR: Oral contraceptives and blood pressure. Arch Intern Med 1969;123:362-365.

226. Lanier AP et al.: Cancer and stilbestrol: A follow-up of 1,719 persons exposed to estrogen *in utero* and born 1943-1959. Mayo Clinic Pro 1973;48:793-799.

227. LaRosa JC: Atherosclerotic risk factors in cardiovascular disease. J Reprod Med 1986;31(9 Suppl):906-912.

228. Laumas KR et al.: Radioactivity in the breastmilk of lactating women after oral administration of 3 H-norethynodrel. Am J Obstet Gynecol 1967;98:411-413.

229. Legler UF: Lack of impairment of fluocortolone disposition in oral contraceptive users. Europ J Clin Pharm 1988;35:101-103.

230. Lesko SM et al.: Evidence for an increased risk of Crohn's disease in oral contraceptive users. Gastroenterology 1985;89(5):1046-1049.

231. Levy EP, Cohen A, Fraser FC: Hormone treatment during pregnancy and congenital heart defects. Lancet 1973;1:611.

232. Lewis JH, Tice HL, Zimmerman HJ: Budd-Chiari syndrome associated with oral contraceptive steroids: Review of treatment of 47 cases. Dig Dis Sci 1983;28(8):673-683.

233. Lewis M, Spitzer WO, Heinemann LAJ, et al.: Lowered risk of dying of heart attack with third-generation contraceptives may offset risk of dying of thromboembolism. Br Med J 1997;315:679-680.

234. Lewis MA, Heinemann LAJ, MacRae KD, Bruppacher R, Spitzer WO: The increased risk of venous thromboembolism and the use of third-generation progestogens: Role of bias in observational research. Contraception 1996;54:5-13.

235. Lewis MA, Heinemann LAJ, Spitzer WO, MacRae KD, Bruppacher R: The use of oral contraceptives and the occurrence of acute myocardial infarction in young women. Contraception 1997;56:129-140.

236. Lewis MA, Spitzer WO, Heinemann LAJ, MacRae KD, Bruppacher R, Thorogood M: Third-generation oral contraceptives and risk of myocardial infarction: An international case-control study. BMJ 1996;312:88-90.

237. Liang MH et al.: Oral estrogen use, menopausal status, and relationship to rheumatoid arthritis. Ann Rheum Dis 1984;43:115.

238. Lidegaard O: Oral contraception and risk of a cerebral thromboembolic attack: Result of a case control study. British Med Journal 1993;306:956-963.

239. Lidegaard O: Oral contraceptives, pregnancy, and the risk of cerebral thromboembolism: The influence of diabetes, hypertension, migraine, and previous thrombotic disease. Br J Obstet Gynaecol 1995;102:153-159.

240. Lindsay R et al.: The effect of oral contraceptive use on vertebral bone mass in pre- and postmenopausal women. Contraception 1986;34:333.

241. Linn S et al.: Lack of association between contraceptive usage and congenital malformations in offspring. Am J Obstet Gynecol 1983; 147(8)923-928.

242. Linos A et al.: Rheumatoid arthritis and oral contraceptives. Lancet 1978;2:871.

243. LiVolsi VA et al.: Fibrocystic disease in oral contraceptive users. N Engl J Med 1977;299:381.

244. Longnecker MP et al.: A meta-analysis of alcohol consumption in relation to risk of breast cancer. JAMA 1988;260:652-656.

245. Longstretch WT, Nelson LM, Koepsell TD, van Belle G: Subarachnoid hemorrhage and hormonal factors in women: A population-based, case control study. Ann Intern Med 1994;121:168-173.

246. Loriaux L, Wild RA: Contraceptive choices for women with endocrine disorders. Am J Obstet Gynecol 1993;168:2021-2026.

247. Luyckx AS et al.: Carbohydrate metabolism in women who used oral contraceptives containing levonorgestrel or desogestrel: A six-month prospective study. Fertil Steril 1986;45(5):635-642.

248. Mack TN et al.: Estrogens and endometrial cancer in a retirement community. N Engl J Med 1976;294:1262-1267.

249. Madhavapeddi R, Ramachandran P: Side effects of oral contraceptive use in lactating women: Enlargement of breast in a breastfed child. Contraception 1985;32(5):437-443.

250. Magidor S et al.: Long-term follow-up of children whose mothers used oral contraceptives prior to conception. Contraception 1984;29(3):203-204.

251. Maguire MG et al.: Increased risk of thrombosis due to oral contraceptives: A further report. Am J Epidemiol 1979;110(2):188-195.

252. Mann JI, Inman WHW: Oral contraceptives and death from myocardial infarction. Br Med J 1975;2:245-248.

253. Mann JI, Inman WHW, Thorogood M: Oral contraceptive use in older women and fatal myocardial infarction. Br Med J 1976;2:445-447.

254. Mann JI et al.: Myocardial infarction in young women with special reference to oral contraceptive practice. Br Med J 1975;2:241-245.

255. Mann JI et al.: Oral contraceptives and myocardial infarction in young women: A further report. Br Med J 1975;2:631-632.

256. Mason B, Oakley N, Wynn V: Studies of carbohydrate and lipid metabolism in women developing hypertension on oral contraceptives. Br Med J 1973;3:317-320.

257. Matthews PN, Millis RR, Hayward VL: Breast cancer in women who have taken contraceptive steroids. Br Med J 1981;282:774.

258. Mattson RH, Cramer JC: Epilepsy, sex hormones, and anti-epileptic drugs. Epilepsia 1985;26:S40-S41.

259. Mattson RH, Cramer JA, Caldwell BV, Siconolfi BC: Treatment of seizures with medroxyprogesterone acetate: Preliminary report. Neurology 1984;34:1255-1258.

260. Mattson RH, Cramer JC, Darney PC, et al.: Use of oral contraceptives by women with epilepsy. JAMA 1986;256:238-240.

261. Mattson RH, Rebar RW: Contraceptive methods for women with neurologic disorders. Am J Obstet Gynecol 1993;168:2027-2032.

262. Mays ET et al.: Hepatic changes in young women ingesting contraceptive steroids: Hepatic hemorrhage and primary hepatic tumors. JAMA 1976;235:730-732.

263. McCredie J et al.: Congenital limb defects and the pill (letter). Lancet 1983;2(8350):623.

264. McGregor JA, Hammill HA: Contraceptive and sexually transmitted disease: Interactions and opportunities. Am J Obstet Gynecol 1993;168:2033-2041.

265. McPherson K et al.: Early oral contraceptive use and breast cancer: The results of another case control study. Br J Cancer 1987;56:653.

266. McPherson K et al.: Oral contraceptives and breast cancer (letter). Lancet 1983;2:1414-1415.

267. Meade TW, Greenberg G, Thompson SF: Progestogens and cardiovascular reactions associated with oral contraceptives and a comparison of the safety of 50 and 30 mg oestrogen preparations. Br Med J 1980;280:1157.

268. Medical Letter. 1981;23:5(578):17-28.
269. Mestman JH, Schmidt-Sarosi C: Diabetes mellitus and fertility control: Contraception management issues. Am J Obstet Gynecol 1993;168:2012-1020.
270. Miller DR et al.: Breast cancer before age 45 and oral contraceptive use: New findings. Am J Epidemiol 1989;129:269-280.
271. Miller DR et al.: Breast cancer risk in relation to early oral contraceptive use. Obstet Gynecol 1986;68:863-868.
272. Miller NE et al.: Relation of angiographically defined coronary artery disease to plasma lipoprotein subfractions and apolipoproteins. Br Med J 1981;282:1741.
273. Mills A: Combined oral contraception and the risk of venous thromboembolism. Hum Repro 1997;12:2595-2598.
274. Milsom I, Andersch B: Effect of various oral contraceptive combinations on dysmenorrhea. Gynecol Obstet Invest 1984;17(6):284-292.
275. Mitchell MC, Hanew T, Meredith CG, Schenker S: Effects of oral contraceptive steroids on acetaminophen metabolism and elimination. Clin Pharm Ther 1983;34:41-53.
276. Moghissi KS: Oral contraceptives and endometrial, cervical, and breast cancers. Ch. 28. In: *Human Reproduction, Conception, and Contraception*, 2nd ed. Hafez ESE (ed.) Hagerstown, PA: Harper and Row, 1978.
277. Mol BWJ, Ankum WM, Bossuyt PMM, Van der Veen F: Contraception and the risk of ectopic pregnancy: A meta-analysis. Contraception 1995;52:337-341.
278. Morris JM, Van Wagenen G: Interception: The use of postovulatory estrogens to prevent implantation. Am J Obstet Gynecol 1973;115:101-106.

279. Mostad SB, Overbaugh J, DeVange DM, Welch MJ, Chohan B, Mandaliya K, Nyange P, Martin HL, Ndinya-Achola J, Bwayo JJ, Kreiss JK: Hormonal contraception, vitamin A deficiency, and risk factors for shedding of HIV-1 infected cells from the cervix and vagina. Lancet 1997;350:922-927.

280. Munroe JS: Progesterone as immunosuppressive agents. J Reticuloendothelial Soc 1971;9:361.

281. Murthy PBK, Prema K: Further studies on sister-chromatid exchange frequency in users of hormonal contraceptives. Mutat Res 1983;119(3):351-354.

282. Myles JL, Hart WR: Apoplectic leiomyomas of the uterus: A clinicopathologic study of five distinctive hemorrhagic leiomyomas associated with oral contraceptive usage. Am J Surg Pathol 1985;9(11):798-805.

283. Nathan B, Evans G, McKeever J: Practice in prescribing emergency contraceptives in A and E departments varies. Br Med J 1998;316:148-149.

284. National Institute of Neurological Disorders and Stroke rt-PA Stroke Study Group. Tissue plasminogen activator for acute ischemic stroke. N Engl J Med 1995;333:1581-1587.

285. Nattero G: Menstrual headache. Adv Neurol 1982;33:215-226.

286. Neuberger J et al.: Oral contraceptive-associated liver tumors: Occurrence of malignancy and difficulties in diagnosis. Lancet 1980;1:273.

287. Neuberger J et al.: Oral contraceptives and hepatocellular carcinoma. Br Med J 1986;292:1355-1357.

288. Newton J et al.: Oral contraceptives and hepatocellular carcinoma. Br Med J (Clin Res) 1986;292:1392.

289. Nissen ED, Kent DR, Nissen SE: Etiologic factors in the pathogenesis of liver tumors associated with oral contraceptives. Am J Obstet Gynecol 1977;127:61.

290. Nisson S, Nygren KG: Transfer of contraceptive steroids to human milk. Res in Reprod 1979;11:1.

291. Nora AH, Nora JJ: A syndrome of multiple congenital anomalies associated with teratogenic exposure. Arch Environmental Health 1975;30:17.

292. Nora JJ, Nora AH: Birth defects and oral contraceptives. Lancet 1973;1:941-942.

293. Norris LA, Bonnar J: The effect of oestrogen dose and progestogen type on haemostatic changes in women taking low-dose oral contraceptives. Br J Obstet Gynecol 1996;103:261-267.

294. Northmann VJ, Chittinand S, Schuster MN: Reversible mesenteric vascular occlusion associated with oral contraceptives. Am J Digestive Dis 1973;18:361.

295. Oakley D: Birth control, emergency contraception still need attention. Fam Plann Perspect 1997;28:277-279.

296. Oberti C et al.: Low dosage oral progestogens to control fertility: Morphologic modifications in the gonad and oviduct. Obstet Gynecol 1974;43:285.

297. *Obstetrician's and Gynecologist's Compendium of Drug Therapy.* New York: Biomedical Information Corporation, 1981-1982;22:7.

298. Ochs HR, Greenblatt DJ, Friedman H, Burstein ES, Locniskz BS, et al.: Bromazepam pharmacokinetics: Influence of age, gender, oral contraceptives, cimetidine, and propranolol. Clin Pharm Ther 1987;41:562-570.

299. Ochs HR, Greenblatt DJ, Verburg-Ochs B, Harmatz JS, Grehl H: Disposition of clotiazepam: Influence of age, sex, oral contraceptives, crimetidine, isoniazid, and ethanol. Europ J Clin Pharm 1984;26:55-59.

300. op ten Berg, M: Desogestrel: Using a selective progestogen in a combined oral contraceptive. Advances In Contraception 1991;7:241-250.

301. Orme MLE, Back DJ, Breckenridge M: Clinical pharmacokinetics of oral contraceptive steroids. Clin Pharm 1983;8:95-136.

302. Orme M, Back DJ, Ward S, et al.: The pharmacokinetics of ethinyl estradiol in the presence and absence of gestodene and desogestrel. Contraception 1991;43:305-316.

303. Ory HW: Health effects of fertility control. In: Contraception: Science, Technology, and Application: Proceedings of a Symposium. Washington, DC: National Academy of Sciences, 1979;110-121.

304. Ory HW: The noncontraceptive health benefits from oral contraceptive use. Fam Plann Perspect 1982;14:182.

305. Ory HW: Oral contraceptive use and breast diseases. In: *Pharmacology of Steroid Contraceptive Drugs.* Garattini S, Berendes HW (ed.) New York: Raven Press, 1977;179-183.

306. Ory HW and the Women's Health Study: Ectopic pregnancy and intrauterine contraceptive devices. Am J Obstet Gynecol 1981;57:137.

307. Ory HW et al.: The effect of a biodegradable contraceptive capsule (Capronor®) containing levonorgestrel on gonadotropin, estrogen, and progesterone levels. Am J Obstet Gynecol 1983;145(5):600-605.

308. Ory HW et al.: Oral contraceptives and reduced risk of benign breast diseases. N Engl J Med 1976;294:419-422.

309. Palatsi R, Hirvensalo E, Liukko P, et al.: Serum total and unbound testosterone and sex hormone binding globulin (SHBG) in female acne patients treated with two different oral contraceptives. Acta Derm Venereol (Stockh) 1984;64(6):517-523.

310. Pardthaisong T, Gray RH: *In utero* exposure to steroid contraceptives and outcome of pregnancy. Am J Epidermiol 1991;134:795-803.

311. Pardthaisong T, Gray RH: The return of fertility following discontinuance of oral contraceptives in Thailand. Fertil Steril 1981;35:532.

312. Pardthaisong T, Gray RH, McDaniel EB, Chandacham A: Steroid contraceptive use and pregnancy outcome. Teratology 1988;38:51-58.

313. Paul C et al.: Oral contraceptives and breast cancer: A national study. Br Med J 1986;293:723-726.

314. Peddie BA et al.: Relationship between contraceptive method and vaginal flora. Austral NZ J Ob Gyn 1984;24:217.

315. Peterson HB et al.: Mortality risk associated with tubal sterilization in the United States. Am J Obstet Gynecol 1982;143:125.

316. Petitti D, Wingerd J: Use of oral contraceptives, cigarette smoking, and risk of subarachnoid hemorrhage. Lancet 1978;2:234-236.

317. Petitti D et al.: Risk of vascular disease in women: Smoking, oral contraceptives, noncontraceptive estrogens, and other factors. JAMA 1979;242(11):1150-1154.

318. Petitti DB, Porterfield D: Worldwide variations in the lifetime probablity of reproductive cancer in women: Implications of best case and worst case assumptions about the effect of oral contraceptive use. Contraception 1992;45:93-104.

319. Petitti DB, Sidney S, Bernstein A, Wolf S, Quesenberry C, Ziel HK: Stroke in users of low-dose oral contraceptives. N Engl J Med 1996;335:8-15.

320. Phillips et al.: Comprehensive comparison of the potencies and activities of progestogens used in contraceptives. Contraception 1987;36:181.

321. Phillips A et al.: Progestational and androgenic receptor binding affinities and in vitro activities of norgestimate and other progestins. Contraception 1990;41:399-410.

322. Physician's Desk Reference, 35th ed. Oradell, NJ: Medical Economics Company, 1981;606.

323. Pike MC et al.: Breast cancer in young women and use of oral contraceptives: Possible modifying effect of formulation and age at use. Lancet 1983;2:926-929.

324. Pike MC et al.: Oral contraceptive use and early abortion as risk factors for breast cancer in young women. Br J Cancer 1981;43:72-76.

325. Piper JM: Oral contraceptives and cervical cancer. Gynecol Oncol 1985;22(1):1-14.

326. Pituitary Adenoma Study Group. Pituitary adenomas and oral contraceptives: A multicenter case control study. Fertil Steril 1983;39(6):753-760.

327. Planned Parenthood Federation of America: Manual of Medical Standards and Guidelines. New York, Planned Parenthood Federation, 1980, Section III-H:29.

328. Polednak AP: Exogenous female sex hormones and birth defects. Pub Health Rev 1985;13(1-2):89-114.

329. Population Information Program. Population Reports. Series A, No. 2, 1975; Series H, No. 2, May 1974; Series I, No. 1, June 1974; Series B, No. 2, January 1976. Washington, DC: George Washington University Medical Center.

330. Porter JB, Hershel J, Walker AM: Mortality among oral contraceptive users. Obstet Gynecol 1987;70:29-32.

331. Porter JB et al.: Oral contraceptives and nonfatal vascular disease. Obstet Gynecol 1985;66:1-4.

332. Potts JC, Papernik E: Mifepristone teratogenicity. Lancet 1991;338:1332-1333.

333. Pye RJ et al.: Effect of oral contraceptives on sebum excretion rate. Br Med J 1977;2:1581-1582.

334. Ramcharan S, Pellegrin FA, Ray RM, Hsu JP: The Walnut Creek Contraceptive Drug Study: A prospective study of the side effects of oral contraceptives. J Reprod Med 1980;25:345-372.

335. Rautio A: Liver function and medroxyprogesterone acetate elimination in man. Biomed and Pharmacother 1984;38:199.

336. Realini JP, Goldzieher JW: Oral contraceptives and cardiovascular disease: A critique of the epidemiologic studies. Am J Obstet Gynecol 1985;152(6, Part 2):729-798.

337. Redmond GP, Olson WH, Lippman JS, Kafrissen ME, Jones TM, Jorizzo JL: Norgestimate and ethinyl estradiol in the treatment of acne vulgaris: A randomized, placebo controlled trial. Obstet Gynecol 1997;89:615-622.

338. Reijnen HBM, Atsma WJ: Risk is highest during first months of use. Br Med J 1995;311:1639.

339. Rhodes JM et al.: Colonic Crohn's disease and use of oral contraception. Br Med J (Clin Res) 1984;288(6417):595-596.

340. Rodin A et al.: Combined oral contraception and skeletal bone mass. Bone 1987;8:53.

341. Rogers SM, Back, Stevenson PJ, Grimmer SFM, Orme ML: Paracetamol interaction with oral contraceptive steroids: Increased plasma concentrations of ethinyl oestradiol. Br J Clin Pharm 1987;23:721-725.

342. Rojanasakul A et al.: Effects of combined desogestrel/ethinyl estradiol treatment on lipid profiles in women with polycystic ovarian disease. Fertil Steril 1987;48(4):581-585.

343. Rooks JB et al.: Epidemiology of hepatocellular adenoma: The role of oral contraceptive use. JAMA 1979;242(7):644-648.

344. Rookus MA, van Leeuwen FE: Oral contraceptives and risk of breast cancer in women aged 20 to 54 years. Lancet 1994;344:844-851.

345. Rosenberg L, Miller DR, Kaufman DW: Breast cancer and oral contraceptive use. Am J Epidemiol 1984;119:167-176.

346. Rosenberg L, Palmer JR, Lesko SM, Shapiro S: Oral contraceptive use and the risk of myocardial infarction. Am J Epidemiol 1991;131:1009-1016.

347. Rosenberg L, Palmer JR, Sands MI, Grimes D, Bergman U, Daling J, Mills A: Modern oral contraceptives and cardiovascular disease. Am J Obstet Gynecol 1997;177:707-715.

348. Rosenberg L, Shapiro S, Slone D: Epithelial ovarian cancer and combination oral contraceptives. JAMA 1982;247:3210-3212.

349. Rosenberg MJ, Waugh MS, Stevens CM: Smoking and cycle control among oral contraceptive users. Am J Obstet Gynceol 1996;174:628-632.

350. Rosing J, Trans G, Nicolaes GAF, et al.: Oral contraceptives and venous thrombosis: Different sensitivities to activated protein C in women using second- and third-generation oral contraceptives. Br J Haematol 1997;97:233-238.

351. Rosner D, Lane WW: Oral contraceptive use has no adverse effect on the prognosis of breast cancer. Cancer 1986;57(3):591-596.

352. Rothman KV, Lovik C: Oral contraceptives and birth defects. N Engl J Med 1978;299:522-524.

353. Roy S et al.: The metabolic effects of a low-estrogen/low-progestogen oral contraceptive: Proceedings of a symposium. New York: Biomedical Information Corporation, 1981;24.

354. Royal College of General Practitioners. Incidence of arterial disease among oral contraceptive users. J Coll Gen Pract 1983;33:75-82.

355. Royal College of General Practitioners. Oral contraception and thromboembolic disease. J Coll Gen Pract 1967;13:267-279.

356. Royal College of General Practitioners. Oral contraceptives and health: An interim report from the oral contraception study of the Royal College of General Practitioners. New York: Pitman, 1974.

357. Royal College of General Practitioners. Oral contraceptives, venous thrombosis, and varicose veins. J Coll Gen Pract 1978;28:393.

358. Royal College of General Practitioners Oral Contraceptive Study. Effect on hypertension and benign breast disease of progestogen component in combined oral contraceptives. Lancet 1977;1:624.

359. Royal College of General Practitioners Oral Contraceptive Study. Further analysis of mortality in oral contraceptive users. Lancet 1981;1:541.

360. Royal College of General Practitioners Oral Contraceptive Study. Reduction in incidence of rheumatoid arthritis associated with oral contraceptives. Lancet 1978;1:569.

361. Russell-Briefel R, Ezzati TM, Perlman JA, Marphy RS: Impaired glucose tolerance in women using oral contraceptives: United States, 1976-1980. J Chronic Dis 1987;40:3-11.

362. Russell-Briefel R et al.: Cardiovascular risk status and oral contraceptive use: United States, 1976-1980. Prev Med 1986;15(4):352-362.

363. Sandmire HF, Austin SD, Bechtel RC: Carcinoma of the cervix in oral contraceptive steroid and IUD users and nonusers. Am J Obstet Gynecol 1976;125:339.

364. Sanhueza H et al.: A randomized double-blind study of two oral contraceptives. Contraception 1979;20:29.

365. Sartwell PE et al.: Thromboembolism and oral contraceptives: An epidemiological case control study. Am J Epidemiol 1969;90:365-380.

366. Schirm A et al.: Contraceptive failure in the U.S.: Importance of social, economic, and demographic factors. Fam Plann Perspect 1982;14:68.

367. Schlesselman J et al.: Breast cancer in relation to early use of oral contraceptives. JAMA 1988;259:1828-1833.

368. Schlesselman JJ: Net effect of oral contraceptive use on the risk of cancer in women in the United States. Obstet Gynecol 1995;85:793-801.

369. Schlesselman JJ: Risk of endometrial cancer in relation to use of combined oral contraceptives: A practitioner's guide to meta-analysis. Hum Reprod 1997;12:1851-1863.

370. Schlesselman JJ et al.: Breast cancer risk in relation to type of estrogen contained in oral contraceptives. Contraception 1988;36:595.

371. Schwallie PC, Assenzo JH: Contraceptive use-efficacy study utilizing medroxyprogesterone acetate administered as an intramuscular injection once every 90 days. Fertil Steril 1973;24:331-339.

372. Scotlenfeld D, Engle RL Jr: Decreased risk of endometrial cancer among oral contraceptive users. N Engl J Med 1980;303:1045.

373. Scragg RK, McMichael AJ, Seamark RF: Oral contraceptives, pregnancy, and endogenous oestrogen in gallstone disease: A case control study. Br Med J (Clin Res) 1984;288(6433): 1795-1799.

374. Senanayake P, Kramer DG: Contraception and the etiology of PID: New perspectives. Am J Obstet Gynecol 1980;138:852-860.

375. Shenfield GM, Griffin JM: Clinical pharmacokinetics of contraceptive steroids. Clinical Pharmacokinetic 1991;(I)20:15-37.

376. Sherman AL et al.: Cervical-vaginal adenosis after *in utero* exposure to synthetic estrogens. Obstet Gynecol 1974;44:531-545.

377. Shikary ZK, Betrabet SS, Patel ZM, et al.: Transfer of LNG administered through different drug delivery systems from the maternal circulation into newborn infant's circulation. Contraception 1987; 35:477-486.

378. Shoupe D: Effects of oral contraceptives on the borderline NIDD patient. Int J Fertil 1991;36:80-86.

379. Shoupe D, Kjos S: Effects of oral contraceptives on the borderline NIDD patient. Int J Fertil 1988;33:27-34.

380. Siegberg R et al.: Sex hormone profiles in oligomenorrheic adolescent girls and the effect of contraceptives. Fertil Steril 1984;41(6):888-893.

381. Silverberg SG, Makowski EL: Endometrial carcinoma in young women taking oral contraceptive agents. Am J Obstet Gyencol 1975;46:503-506.

382. Silverberg SG, Makowski EL, Roche WD: Endometrial carcinoma in women under 40 years of age: Comparisons of cases in oral contraceptive users and nonusers. Cancer 1977;39:592-598.

383. Sidney S, Petitti DB, Quesenberry CP, Klatsky AL, Wolf S: Myocardial infarction in users of low-dose oral contraceptives. Obstet Gynecol 1996;88:939-944.

384. Sivin I: International experience with Norplant® and Norplant-2® contraceptives. Stud Fam Plann 1988;19:81-94.

385. Skouby SO, Molsted-Pedersen L, Kuhl C, Bennet P: Oral contraceptives in diabetic women: Metabolic effects of four compounds with different estrogen/progestogen profiles. Fertil Steril 1986;46:858-864.

386. Skouby SO, Molsted-Pedersen L, Peterson KR: Contraception for women with diabetes: An update. Clin Obstet Gynecol 1991;5:493-503.

387. Slone D, Shapiro S, Kaufman DW: Risk of myocardial infarction in relation to current and discontinued use of oral contraceptives. N Engl J Med 1981;305:420-424.

388. Smith DC et al.: Association of exogenous estrogen and endometrial carcinoma. N Engl J Med 1975;293:1164-1167.

389. Souka AR et al.: Vaginal administration of a combined oral contraceptive containing norethisterone acetate. Contraception 1985; 31(6):571-581.

390. Spanos WJ: Preoperative hormonal therapy of cystic adnexal masses. Am J Obstet Gynecol 1973;116:551.

391. Sparrow MJ: Pill method failures. New Zealand Med J 1987;100:102-105.

392. Sparrow MJ: Pregnancies in reliable pill takers. New Zealand Med J 1989;102:575-577.

393. Spellacy WN, Birk SA: The development of elevated blood pressure while using oral contraceptives: A preliminary report of a prospective study. Fertil Steril 1970;21:301-306.

394. Speroff L, DeCherney A, et al.: Evaluation of a new generation of oral contraceptives. Obstet Gynecol 1993;81:1034-1047.

395. Spitzer WO: The 1995 pill scare revisited: Anatomy of a nonepidemic. Hum Reprod 1997;12:2347-1357.

396. Spitzer WO, Lewis MA, Heinemann LAJ, Thorogood M, MacRae KD: Third-generation oral contraceptives and risk of venous thromboembolic disorders: An international case control study. BMJ 1996;312:83-87.

397. Spona J, Elstein M, Feichtinger W, Sullivan H, Ludicke F, Muller U, Dusterberg B: Shorter pill-free interval in combined oral contraceptives decreases follicular development. Contraception 1996;54:71-77.

398. Stadel BV, Schlesselman JJ: Oral contraceptive use and the risk of breast cancer in women with a prior history of benign breast disease. Am J Epidemiol 1986;123(3):373-382.

399. Staffa JA, Newschaffer CJ, Jones JK, Miller V: Progestins and breast cancer: An epidemiologic review. Fertil Steril 1992;57:473-491.

400. Stafi A et al.: Clinical diagnosis of vaginal adenosis. Obstet Gynecol 1974;43:118-128.

401. Stanford JL: Oral contraceptives and neoplasia of the ovary. Contraception 1991;43:543-556.

402. Steinberger E et al.: Testosterone, DHEA, and DHEA sulfate in hyperandrogenic women. J Clin Endo Metab 1984;59:471.

403. Stewart WF, Lipton RB, Celentano DD, Reed ML: Prevalence of migraine headache in the United States: Relation to age, income, race, and other sociodemographic factors. JAMA 1992;267:64-69.

404. Stolley PD et al.: Thrombosis with low-estrogen oral contraceptives. Am J Epidemiol 1975;102:197-208.

405. Strom BL et al.: Oral contraceptives and other risk factors for gallbladder disease. Clin Pharmacol Ther 1986;39(3):335-341.

406. Stumpf PG: Selecting constant serum estradiol levels achieved by vaginal rings. Obstet Gynecol 1986;57:91-94.

407. Suissa S, Blais L, Spitzer WO, Cusson J: First-time use of newer oral contraceptives and the risk of venous thromboembolism. Contraception 1997;56:128-132.

408. Su-Juan GU, Ming-Kun DU, Ling-De Z, Ying-Lin LIU, Shu-Hua W, Sivin I: A five-year evaluation of Norplant® contraceptive implants in China. Obstet Gynecol 1994;83:673-678.

409. Sullivan JM, Lobo RA: Considerations for contraception in women with cardiovascular disorders. Am J. Obstet Gynecol 1993;168:2006-2011.

410. Surveillance, Epidemiology and End Results. Incidence and Mortality Data 1973-77. National Cancer Institute Monograph 57, June 1981. (NIH publication No. 81-2330).

411. Svensson L, Westrom L, Mardh PA: Contraceptives and acute salpingitis. JAMA 1984;251:2553-2555.

412. Svensson PJ, Dahlback B: Resistance to activated protein C as a basis for venous thrombosis. New Engl J Med 330:517-522.

413. Swyer GIM: Oral contraceptives and cancer. Lancet 1983;2:1019.

414. Swyer GIM, Little V: Clinical assessment of orally active progestogens. Proc R Soc Med 1962;55:861-868.

415. Swyer GIM, Little V: Clinical assessment of relative potency of progestogens. J Repro Fertil 1968;5(suppl):63-68.

416. Swyer GIM, Little V: Potency of progestogens and oral contraceptives: Further delay-of-menses data. Contraception 1982;26:23.

417. Symposia Reporter. 1989 Consensus Conference on Sex Hormones in Women, October 1989. Co-chairmen: Leon Speroff, John C. Larosa.

418. Szabo AG, Cole HS, Grimaldi RD: Glucose tolerance in gestational diabetic women during and after treatment with the combination type oral contraceptives. N Engl J Med 1970;282:646.

419. Talwar PP, Berger GS: Side effects of drugs: The relation of body weight to side effects associated with oral contraceptives. Br Med J 1977;1:1637-1638.

420. Tankeyoon M et al.: Effects of hormonal contraceptives on milk volume and infant growth: WHO Special Programme of Research, Development, and Research Training in Human Reproduction. Contraception 1984;30(6):505-522.

421. Task Force on Oral Contraceptives. A randomized, double-blind study of the effects of two low-dose combined oral contraceptives on biochemical aspects: Report from a seven-centered study. WHO Special Programme of Research, Development, and Research Training in Human Reproduction. Contraception 1985;32(3):223-236.

422. Tausk M, de Visser J: International Encyclopedia of Pharmacology and Therapeutics. Ch. 28, Sect. 48, Vol. II. Elmsford, NY: Pergamon Press, 1972.

423. Thau RB: Luteinizing hormone-releasing hormone (LHRH) and its analogs for contraception in women: A review. Contraception 1984;29(2):143-162.

424. Thomas DB: The WHO collaborative study of neoplasia and steroid contraceptives: The influence of combined oral contraceptives or risk of neoplasms in developing and developed countries. Contraception 1991;43:695-710.

425. Thomas SHL: Mortality from venous thromboembolism and myocardial infarction in young adults in England and Wales. Lancet 1996;348:402.

426. Thomsen RJ: Utilization of Norplant® subdermal contraceptive devices. Clin Obstet 1985; 23(3):223-227.

427. Thorogood M, Mann J, Murphy M, Vessey M: Fatal stroke and use of oral contraceptives: Findings from a case control study. Am J Epidemiol 1992;136:35-45.

428. Thorogood M, Mann J, Murphy M, Vessey M: Is oral contraceptive use still associated with an increased risk of fatal myocardial infarction? Br J Obstet Gynaecol 1991;98:1245-1253.

429. Tietze C: New estimates of mortality associated with fertility control. Fam Plann Perspect 1977; 9(2):74-76.

430. Tietze C, Bongaarts V, Schearer B: Mortality associated with the control of fertility. Fam Plann Perspect 1976;8:6-14.

431. TIMI [Thrombosis in Myocardial Infarction] Study Group. The thrombolisis in myocardial infarction (TIMI) trial, Phase I findings. N Engl J Med 1985;312:932-936.

432. Toddywalla VS, Patel SB, Betrabet SS, Kulkarni RD, Saxena BN: Is time-interval between mini-pill ingestion and breastfeeding essential? Contraception 1995;51:192-205.

433. Trussell J, Hatcher RA, Cates W Jr., Stewart FH, Kost K: A guide to interpreting contraceptive efficacy studies. Obstet Gynecol 1990;76:558-567.

434. Trussell J, Kost K: Contraceptive failure in the United States: A critical review of the literature. Stud Fam Plann 1987;18(5):237-283.

435. Tyrer LB: Oral contraception for the adolescent. J Repro Med 1984;29(7suppl):551-559.

436. Tyrer LB: Suggested patient instruction concerning missed pills. Memorandum. New York: Planned Parenthood Federation of America, August 3, 1976.

437. UK National Case Control Study Group. Oral contraceptive use and breast cancer risk in young women: Subgroup analyses. Lancet 1990; 335:1507-1509.

438. Ursin G, Peters RK, Henderson BE, d'Ablaing G, Monroe KR, Pike MC: Oral contraceptive use and adenocarcinoma of cervix. Lancet 1994;344:1390-1394.

439. U.S. Food and Drug Administration. Oral contraceptive labeling. Washington, DC: U.S. Government Printing Office, 1980.

440. U.S. Food and Drug Administration. Oral contraceptives and cancer. FDA Drug Bulletin 1984;14(1):2-3.

441. Valente PT, Hanjani P: Endocervical neoplasia in long-term users of oral contraceptives: Clinical and pathologic observations. Obstet Gynecol 1986;67:695-704.

442. Valla D et al.: Risk of hepatic vein thrombosis in relation to recent use of oral contraceptives: A case-control study. Gastroenterology 1986; 90(4):807-811.

443. Vandenbroucke JP, Helmerhorst FM, Bloemenkamp KWM, Rosendaal FR: Third-generation oral contraceptive and deep venous thrombosis: From epidemiologic controversy to new insight in coagulation. Am J Obstet Gynecol 1997;177:887-891.

444. Vandenbrouke JP, Koster T, Briet E, et al.: Increased risk of venous thrombosis in oral contraceptive users who are carriers of factor V Leiden mutation. Lancet 1994:344:1453-1457.

445. Vandenbroucke JP et al.: Noncontraceptive hormones and rheumatoid arthritis in premenopausal and postmenopausal women. JAMA 1986;255:1299.

446. Vandenbroucke JP et al.: Oral contraceptives and rheumatoid arthritis: Further evidence for a protective effect. Lancet 1982;2:839-842.

447. Van Deijk WA, Biljham GH, Mellink WAM, Meulenberg PMM: Influence of aminoglutethimide on plasma levels of medroxyprogesterone acetate: Its correlation with serum cortisol. Cancer Treatment Rep. 1985;69:85-90.

448. Van Santen MR, Haspels AA: A comparison of high-dose estrogens vs low-dose ethinyl estradiol and norgestrel combination in postcoital interception: A study in 493 women. Fertil Steril 1985;43(2):206-213.

449. Vekemans M: Use of long-acting contraceptives. Lancet 1995;346:1165.

450. Vessey MP: Female hormones and vascular disease: An epidemiological overview. Br J Fam Plann 1980;6:1-12.

451. Vessey MP: The Jephcott Lecture, 1989: An overview of the benefits and risks of combined oral contraceptives. In: Mann RD, ed. *Oral Contraceptives and Breast Cancer*. Park Ridge, New Jersey: Parthenon 1989;121:35.

452. Vessey MP: Oral contraceptives and breast cancer: Epidemiological evidence. IARC Sci Publ 1985;(65):37-48.

453. Vessey MP, Doll R: Investigation of relation between use of oral contraceptives and thromboembolic disease. Br Med J 1968;2:199-205.

454. Vessey MP, Doll R: Investigation of relation between use of oral contraceptives and thromboembolic disease: A further report. Br Med J 1969;2:651-657.

455. Vessey MP, Doll R, Jones K: Oral contraceptives and breast cancer: Progress report of an epidemiological study. Lancet 1975;1:941-943.

456. Vessey MP, Doll R, Sutton PM: Oral contraceptives and breast neoplasia: A retrospective study. Br Med J 1972;3:719-724.

457. Vessey MP, Lawless M, Yeates D: Oral contraceptives and stroke: Findings in a large prospective study. Br Med J (Clin Res) 1984;289(6444):530-531.

458. Vessey MP, McPherson K, Johnson B: Mortality among women participating in the Oxford Family Planning Association Contraceptive Study. Lancet 1977;2:731-733.

459. Vessey MP, McPherson K, Yeates D: Mortality in oral contraceptive users. Lancet 1981;1:549.

460. Vessey MP, Villard-MacKintosh L, Painter R: Epidemiology of endometriosis in women attending family planning clinics. Br Med J 1993;306:182-184.

461. Vessey MP et al.: A long-term follow-up study of women using different methods of contraception: An interim report. J Biosoc Sci 1976;8:373-427.

462. Vessey MP et al.: An epidemiological study of oral contraceptives and breast cancer. Br Med J 1979;1:1757.

463. Vessey MP et al.: Chronic inflammatory bowel disease, cigarette smoking, and use of oral contraceptives: Findings in a large cohort study of women of childbearing age. Br Med J (Clin Res) 1986;292(6528):1101-1103.

464. Vessey MP et al.: Fertility after stopping different methods of contraception. Br Med J 1978;1:265-267.

465. Vessey MP et al.: Neoplasia of the cervix and uterus and contraception: A possible adverse effect of the pill. Lancet 1983;2:930-934.

466. Vessey MP et al.: Oral contraception and serious psychiatric illness: Absence of an association. Br J Psychiatry 1985;146:45-49.

467. Vessey MP et al.: Oral contraceptive use and abortion before first term pregnancy in relation to breast cancer risk. Br J Cancer 1982;45:327-331.

468. Vessey MP et al.: Oral contraceptives and breast cancer: Final report of an epidemiological study. Br J Cancer 1983;47(4):455-462.

469. Vessey MP et al.: Postoperative thromboembolism and the use of oral contraceptives. Br Med J 1970;3:123-126.

470. Waetjen LE, Grimes DA: Oral contraceptives and primary liver cancer: Temporal trends in three countries. Obstet Gynecol 1996;88:945-949.

471. Wahl P et al.: Effect of estrogen/progestin potency on lipid/lipoprotein cholesterol. N Engl J Med 1983;308:862.

472. Wallace RB et al.: Altered plasma lipid and lipoprotein levels associated with oral contraceptive and oestrogen use. Lancet 1979;2:111-114.

473. Walnut Creek Contraceptive Drug Study. Results of the Walnut Creek Contraceptive Drug Study. J Repro Med 1980;25(suppl):346.

474. Wambach G et al.: Interaction of synthetic progestogens with renal mineral-corticoid receptors. Acta Endocrinol 1979;92(3):560-567.

475. Watson KJR, Ghabrial H, Mashford ML, Harman PJ, Breen KJ, et al.: Effects of sex and the oral contraceptive pill on morphine disposition. Clin Exper Pharmacol Physiol 1987;14:33.

476. Weinstein E, Silverman L: Splenic artery thrombosis secondary to oral contraceptive medication: A case report. Milit Med 1982;147(7):589-590.

477. Weiss NS, Sayvetz TA et al.: Incidence of endometrial cancer in relation to oral contraceptives. N Engl J Med 1980;302:551.

478. Weiss NS et al.: Incidence of ovarian cancer in relation to use of oral contraceptives. Int J Cancer 1981;28:669-671.

479. White E, Malone KE, Weiss NS, Daling JR: Breast cancer among young U.S. women in relation to oral contraceptive use. J Natl Cancer Inst 1994;86:505-514.

480. Wild RA et al.: Hirsutism: Metabolic effects of two commonly used oral contraceptives and spironolactone. Contraception 1991;44:113-124.

481. Wilson ES et al.: A prospective controlled study of the effect on the blood pressure of contraceptive preparations containing different types and dosages of progestogen. Br J Obstet Gynaecol 1984;91(12):1254-1260.

482. Wingrave SJ, Kay CR: Reduction in incidence of rheumatoid arthritis associated with oral contraceptives. Lancet 1978;1:569.

483. Wirth JC, Lohman TG: The relationship of static muscle function to use of oral contraceptives. Med Sci in Sports Exerc 1982;14:16.

484. World Health Organization (WHO): Facts about an implantable contraceptive. Memorandum. Bull WHO 1985;63(3):485-494.

485. World Health Organization (WHO) Collaborative Study of Cardiovascular Disease and Steroid Hormone Contraception. Acute myocardial infarction and combined oral contraceptives: Results of an international multicentre case control study. Lancet 1997;349:1202-1209.

486. World Health Organization (WHO) Collaborative study on cardiovascular disease and steroid hormone contraception. Effect of different progestins in low oestrogen oral contraceptives on venous thromboembolic disease. Lancet 1995; 346:1582-1588.

487. World Health Organizaton (WHO) Collaborative Study of Cardiovascular Disease and Steroid Hormone Contraception. Hemorrhagic stroke, overall stroke risk, and combined oral contraceptives: Results of an international multicentre case control study. Lancet 1996;348:505-510.

488. World Health Organization (WHO) Collaborative Study of Cardiovascular Disease and Steroid Hormone Contraception. Ischemic stroke and combined oral contraceptives: Results of an international multicentre case control study. Lancet 1996;348:498-505.

489. World Health Organization (WHO) Collaborative study on cardiovascular disease and steroid hormone contraception. Venous thromboembolic disease and combined oral contraceptives: Results of international multicentre case control study. Lancet 1995;346:1575-1582.

490. World Health Organization (WHO) Collaborative Study of Neoplasia and Steroid Contraceptives. Breast cancer and depomedroxyprogesterone acetate: A multinational study. Lancet 1991;338:833-838.

491. World Health Organization (WHO) Collaborative Study of Neoplasia and Steroid Contraceptives. Depomedroxyprogesterone acetate (DMPA) and risk of endometrial cancer. Int J Cancer 1991;49:186-190.

492. World Health Organization (WHO) Collaborative Study of Neoplasia and Steroid Contraceptives. Depomedroxyprogesterone acetate (DMPA) and risk of epithelial ovarian cancer. Int J Cancer 1991;49:191-95.

493. World Health Organization (WHO) Collaborative Study of Neoplasia and Steroid Contraceptives. Depomedroxyprogesterone acetate (DMPA) and risk of invasive squamous cell cervical cancer. Contraception 1992;45:299-312.

494. World Health Organization (WHO) Collaborative Study of Neoplasia and Steroid Contraceptives. Depomedroxyprogesterone acetate (DMPA) and risk of liver cancer. Int J Cancer 1991;49:182-85.

495. World Health Organization (WHO) Collaborative Study of Neoplasia and Steroid Contraceptives. Invasive cervical cancer and combined oral contraceptives. Br Med J (Clin Res) 1985;290(6473):961-965.

496. World Health Organization (WHO) Collaborative Study of Neoplasia and Steroid Contraceptives. Invasive cervical cancer and depo-medroxyprogesterone acetate. Bull WHO 1985;63(3):505-511.

497. Wynn V: Effect of duration of low-dose oral contraceptive administration on carbohydrate metabolism. Am J Obstet Gynecol 1982;142:739.

498. Wynn V: Vitamins and oral contraceptive use. Lancet 1975;1:561-564.

499. Wynn V, Doar JWH, Mills GL: Some effects of oral contraceptives on serum lipid and lipoprotein levels. Lancet 1966;2:720-723.

500. Wynn V, Nathyanthas R: The effects of progestins in combined oral contraceptives on serum lipids with special reference to high-density lipoproteins. Am J Obstet Gynecol 1982;142:766.

501. Wynn V et al.: Comparison of effects of different combined oral contraceptive formulations on carbohydrate and lipid metabolism. Lancet 1979;1:1045-1049.

502. Wynn V et al.: Effects of oral contraceptives on carbohydrate metabolism. J Reprod Med 1986;31(9 Suppl):892-897.

503. Wysowski DK, Green L: Serious adverse events in Norplant® users reported to the Food and Drug Administration's MedWatch Spontaneous Reporting System. Obstet Gynecol 1995;85:538-542.

504. Yelland A, Graham MD, Trott PA, Ford HT, Coombes RC, Gazet JC, Polson NG: Diagnosing breast carcinoma in young women. Br Med J 1991;302:618-620.

505. Ylikorkala O: Ovarian cysts and hormonal contraception. Lancet 1977;1:1101-1102.

506. Yuzpe AA, Lancee WJ: Ethinyl estradiol and dl-norgestrel as a postcoital contraceptive. Fertil Steril 1977;28:932.

507. Yuzpe AA, Percival-Smith R, Rademaker AW: A multicenter clinical investigation employing ethinyl estradiol combined with dl-norgestrel as a postcoital contraceptive agent. Fertil Steril 1982;37:508.

508. Zafrani ES, Pinaudeau Y, Dhumeaux D: Drug-induced vascular lesions of the liver. Arch Intern Med 1983;143:495-502.

509. Zafrani ES et al.: Focal hemorrhagic necrosis of the liver. Gastroenterology 1980;79:1295-1299.

510. Ziel HK, Kinkle WD: Increased risk of endometrial carcinoma among users of conjugated estrogens. N Engl J Med 1975;293:1167-1170.